THIRD EDITION

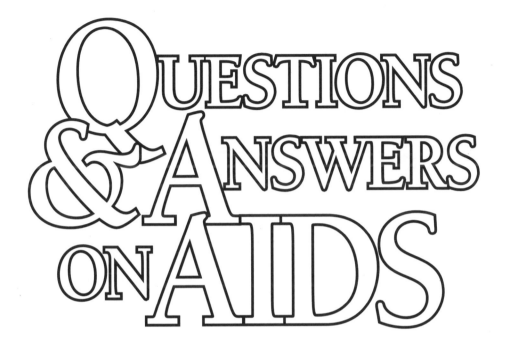

Preface by David D. Ho, M.D.
Forward by Elisabeth Kubler-Ross, M.D.

Lyn R. Frumkin, M.D., Ph.D.
& John M. Leonard, M.D.

HEALTH INFORMATION PRESS
Los Angeles, California 90010

Library of Congress Catalog Number (LCCN): 96-078924

ISBN: 1-885987-07-2

Health Information Press
4727 Wilshire Blvd., Suite 300
Los Angeles, California 90010
(800) MED-SHOP

DEDICATION

To Paul, my nine year-old son, that HIV may be irrelevant.

JML

To the memory of Herbert S. Ripley, M.D., physician, teacher, and friend.

LRF

CONTENTS

CHAPTER THREE
Opportunistic Infections 31

CHAPTER SEVEN

CHAPTER EIGHT
HIV and Public Policy 171

FOREWORD

AIDS first appeared in the United States 15 years ago and, although the significance was not fully appreciated initially, it soon became evident that this disease was more than just a new medical syndrome. As reports of cases accumulated, people began to fear that AIDS was to become one of the greatest national, if not world, health issues of the present time.

Drs. Frumkin and Leonard's third edition of *Questions & Answers on AIDS* continues to be a welcome addition to the ever-increasing literature on AIDS. It remains a meticulous and clearly written collection of the myriad of issues facing this epidemic, addressed not only to caretakers, but also to the healthy infected person, the AIDS patient, and his or her family. In addition to the person with AIDS, those caring for the affected person are also in need of information and an accurate understanding of the illness to best prepare for a lengthy and often lonely vigil at the bedside of a dying adult or child.

This book, which is written in an objective and understandable fashion, should be read by anyone who is afraid of AIDS. All people, whether caretakers or not, need to know that they cannot contract AIDS by casual contact and this book will help them appreciate that. It will also minimize the pathological fear that millions have expressed toward those who have AIDS or are infected with HIV. If individuals can detach themselves from their panic, reading this book may enlighten many people on the subject of AIDS, as well as encourage them to "pitch in" and help their fellow man.

With the rapid increase of AIDS cases within and outside the United States, it is mandatory that we prepare ourselves now and not tomorrow. This can be done, in part, by recruiting a generation of volunteers and health care workers willing to staff hospices for adults and children with this deadly disease. We can also minimize costly hospital stays, which persons with AIDS can least afford, by working to create alternatives for housing those who are not in need of an acute hospital setting. With many AIDS patients currently being cared for in hospital rooms at a cost of $1000/day, such alternatives will slow the financial burden this disease has placed on our health care system.

AIDS is more than just a disease. It is a phenomenon that brings into the open our "dis-ease" —our own fears, prejudices, and need to blame, judge, and criticize others. Although many continue to choose to see AIDS as a disease affecting primarily homosexual men, it is a terminal illness affecting thousands from all walks of life. AIDS is an ultimate challenge to a society rarely faced with a disease that has raised as great a degree of psychological, social, legal, and ethical dilemmas. The fact that AIDS mainly affects young adults and children provokes even more fear and anguish, in proportions far greater than the social turmoil that surrounded the dreaded leprosy of Father Damien's time.

Let your friends and neighbors read this book, and discuss with each other its implications. Make it an issue to share it with your children, so they can too express their feelings and consider accepting a hemophiliac child with AIDS to their classroom and playground. This is your chance to base your understanding and decisions on knowledge and not on fear. I thank Drs. Frumkin and Leonard for sharing this meaningful information with the many who will read it.

Elisabeth Kubler-Ross, M.D.
Scottsdale, Arizona
January 1, 1997

PREFACE

The acquired immunodeficiency syndrome (AIDS) was initially reported in 1981, and its causative agent, the human immunodeficiency virus (HIV), was first identified in 1983. Much has transpired since then. Scientific research has led to unprecedented progress in our understanding of how a virus works, and how this virus in particular destroys a vital component of the immune system. Ten drugs against HIV have been developed and licensed. This arsenal of therapeutics has completely altered the management of infected patients in developed countries, where AIDS is no longer an inevitably fatal disease with no recourse. It is now possible to control the replication of HIV substantially, especially through the use of certain effective drug combinations. There is even a glimmer of hope that someday the virus might be eradicated from an infected person. Better prophylaxis and treatment of a number of AIDS complications has also prolonged the lives of those affected.

Unfortunately, these medical advances have had little impact on the spread of HIV worldwide. The epidemic rages on unperturbed in Africa, Asia and elsewhere. Twenty-three million people have been infected already, and nearly all are doomed to die from this dreadful disease. In the United States, the epidemic has shifted from the male homosexual population into the urban poor. In the absence of a cure or vaccine, efforts to contain the HIV pandemic will largely depend on effective preventive measures that are based on sound information and education.

To that end, everyone should know the fundamentals about HIV and AIDS. Drs. Frumkin and Leonard have done a great service to all by updating their book, *Questions and Answers on AIDS*. Without being overly technical, the book provides important and useful information about the epidemic, the virus, the disease syndrome, and its myriad complications. It explains how HIV is transmitted, and how it isn't transmitted. It contains a practical guide to HIV testing as well. Furthermore, the authors have done an outstanding job of laying down the principles of HIV therapy in keeping with recent advances in our understanding of HIV replication *in vivo* as well as with the growing armamentarium of anti-HIV drugs.

There is no doubt that this book will serve as a valuable tool on HIV/AIDS for patients, family members and friends. Students of all ages will benefit enormously from this practical resource. Knowledge is the power needed to help and to heal. It is also the basis for alleviating unwarranted fear and discrimination.

David D. Ho, M.D.
Director
Aaron Diamond AIDS Research Center
New York, New York
January 1, 1997

A NOTE FROM
THE AUTHORS

The idea to write this book originated from the countless questions posed to us by friends, patients, families of patients, and health professionals during our training as resident physicians at Stanford University Hospital in 1984 and early 1985. The cause of AIDS had recently been discovered, we were caring for patients in an area of the country that was an epicenter for AIDS, and we sensed that the information explosion on this illness was only beginning. In 1986 we believed that there was a lack of easy-to-read, accessible literature that would allow both health care workers and those without medical expertise to acquire general but comprehensive information about AIDS.

We first undertook this project then, during a period when almost daily reports from television and the popular press reflected a need for information on social, ethical, legal and medical aspects of AIDS. Since the publication of our first edition of *Questions & Answers on AIDS* in 1987, the demand for information on HIV and AIDS has substantially increased.

The publication of our second edition of *Questions & Answers on AIDS* coincided with the beginning of the second decade of the AIDS crisis. We retained the question-and-answer format as the best way to balance what we believed was a readable presentation with one sufficiently sophisticated to incorporate both the necessary detail and accuracy. Our goal was to educate the reader by answering questions that routinely arose concerning HIV and AIDS.

Now, as we write this third edition of *Questions and Answers on AIDS*, much has changed once again. The viral cause of AIDS is beyond dispute. Sufficient knowledge has accumulated to permit a very detailed understanding of how HIV grows in the body and why resistance to most therapies often emerges quickly. Simultaneous with a new understanding of how HIV causes disease was the development of a new class of drugs, the protease inhibitors. These drugs, when combined with other compounds from the well-known nucleoside analogue class, produce unprecedented antiviral effects with reductions of HIV in blood to levels that approach zero. This antiviral activity is measured with new techniques called branched DNA (bDNA) and polymerase chain reaction (PCR) that quantitate the amount of virus in blood.

Despite new hope that is truly warranted, many questions central to HIV infection remain unanswered. Worse, the spread of AIDS continues around the world and the new therapies are unattainable for the vast majority of people infected with HIV. By 1994 it was estimated that one in 250 Americans were infected by HIV and estimates are that approximately 40 million people worldwide will have HIV infection by the end of this decade. Much remains to be learned and done before the final word on AIDS is written.

L.R.F
J.M.L.
March 31, 1997

ACKNOWLEDGMENTS

We wish to thank our managing editor, Kathy Swanson, and friends and colleagues who have contributed helpful comments and critical review to past and current editions of this book, including: William Audeh, Ann Collier, Lawrence Corey, Marilyn Foote, Tara Hawkins, Katharine Knowles, William Hanson, Amy Harris-McAferty, R. James Kellogg, Joan C. Leonard, William Lutge, Kenneth Melmon, Gordon Nary, John Sotos, and Shirah Vollmer. At all times they have shared our desire to provide a book that could help the reader to understand better the acquired immunodeficiency syndrome.

INTRODUCTION

In 1981 an epidemic of fatal infections first appeared in homosexual men. The susceptibility to infections in these men resulted from failure of their immune systems to eliminate microorganisms that pose no threat to healthy people. The inability to respond to infection was surprising in that none had any recognized condition known to affect the immune system. What initially seemed to be a condition limited to homosexual men quickly expanded to include intravenous drug users and some recipients of blood transfusions. The spread of this illness to these groups suggested that an infectious agent, transmissible through blood and semen, caused the immune deficiency that was common to all the patients. The term Acquired Immunodeficiency Syndrome, or AIDS, was coined to describe this illness. It had become clear that the infections suffered by these patients were the result of an acquired failure of the immune system that predisposed affected persons to frequent and overwhelming infections. At the outset of the epidemic most people with AIDS died within a year of their diagnosis. In 1983, researchers isolated the virus that causes AIDS. By that time, however, over 12,000 Americans had contracted AIDS and the extent of the epidemic was only beginning to be recognized.

We have learned much about AIDS in the 15 years since the first case reports. We now know that AIDS is caused by human immunodeficiency virus (HIV), its modes of transmission, and who is at risk for HIV infection. We know that HIV kills lymphocytes, cells in the bloodstream necessary to respond to bacteria, fungi, protozoa, and viruses. We have learned that although it is detectable in many body fluids, HIV is transmitted almost exclusively through sexual contact, the sharing of needles used to inject intravenous drugs, and by passage of the virus by an infected mother to her baby at or around the time of birth.

There are millions of people worldwide who are infected with HIV and do not yet have AIDS. We now recognize that AIDS is the most severe manifestation of infection with HIV. We also understand that regardless of the presence of symptoms, each infected person can transmit HIV to others.

Even though much has been learned, people with AIDS still have a poor prognosis. Drugs that are active against HIV have been developed, however they often produce unacceptable side effects and, despite much optimism, as yet have not been shown to cure the infection. Much remains to be learned about HIV infection and its treatment. Nonetheless, it is imperative that we discuss, teach, and study what is already known. Understanding the nature of HIV may help prevent its spread, as well as help lessen the suffering that it causes. It is in the spirit of that understanding that we have written this book.

—CHAPTER ONE—

The Cause Of AIDS

1. What is AIDS?

In 1981 unusual infections were identified in a small number of homosexual men in California and New York. The infections responded poorly to therapy and ended in the death of the patient. Because none of the patients suffered from any condition known to predispose to infections, physicians concluded that the patients had developed an illness never before described in the medical literature. The new condition was named the Acquired Immuno-deficiency Syndrome, or AIDS.

The name *AIDS* acknowledged all of the fundamental characteristics of the illness, in particular the underlying impairment of the immune system and resulting inability to fight infections. The word *acquired* was chosen because the illness was not inherited or the result of other recognized conditions; the illness developed during a period of health with no identifiable explanation for the immunodeficiency. The word *syndrome* signified that the disease could present with many different clinical manifestations but that the affected patients ultimately had the same underlying illness. A syndrome is a constellation of findings that when combined, indicate the presence of a particular illness. For example, persons with AIDS have illnesses that range from cancer in one patient to pneumonia in the next, although in both cases the illnesses occur as the result of the same problem. It became apparent that immune deficiency was the common denominator linking the different illnesses in patients with AIDS.

Several years elapsed between the first reports of AIDS and the identification of the virus that caused it, the human immunodeficiency virus (HIV). The isolation of HIV provided an explanation for the transmission patterns of AIDS as well as the immune deficiency. The name *acquired immunodeficiency syndrome* was selected in 1981 to describe what scientists and the medical community knew about the illness at the time that it was named. The term *AIDS* is now a part of everyday speech.

2. Is AIDS a new illness?

AIDS was unrecognized in organized medicine before it was first reported in 1981. Since the identification of HIV as the cause of AIDS, tests on stored blood found HIV infection in samples from central Africa collected as early as 1959. In other regions, poorly understood cases that occurred years before the AIDS epidemic have now been identified as AIDS, indicating that isolated cases of AIDS occurred in Europe and the United States since the 1960s. The existence of AIDS before the late 1950s is speculative, although it may have existed elsewhere in the world for many years far from the observation of Western physicians. From the perspective of modern medicine, however, AIDS is a newly recognized illness.

Transmissible animal illnesses characterized by severely altered immunity were well known before AIDS appeared in humans. Some of these animal illnesses had been studied for years and provided the impetus to search for a viral cause of AIDS. The spread of AIDS outside the male homosexual population further supported the theory that a transmissible agent caused AIDS. The search for the causative agent culminated in the discovery of a virus in 1983 at the Pasteur Institute in France. The discoverers of this new virus named it *Lymphadenopathy Associated Virus (LAV)*. Shortly after the French discovery, two American laboratories corroborated the initial finding and called their viruses *Human T-cell Lymphotropic Virus III (HTLV-III)* and *AIDS-Associated Retrovirus (ARV)*. An international committee agreed to rename the virus *human immunodeficiency virus (HIV)* in 1987.

3. What is the evidence that HIV causes AIDS?

A substantial body of evidence widely accepted by scientists and physicians alike supports HIV as the causative agent of AIDS. HIV is routinely isolated from individuals who have AIDS and AIDS-related illnesses. Improved virus detection techniques uniformly find HIV in virtually all patients with AIDS. The mere isolation of HIV, however, is not proof that it causes illness. Some have argued that HIV is only a passenger found in the blood and that it does not cause AIDS. Proponents of this theory claim that although HIV is found in patients with AIDS, there are other risk factors, usually either recreational drug use or some other as yet undiscovered factor associated with sexual promiscuity, that are the true cause of AIDS. This argument has lost scientific credibility because of the overwhelming evidence in support of HIV infection as the cause of AIDS. There is no agent other than HIV that even remotely accounts for the patterns of transmission of the disease, the means of disease production (called the pathogenesis of AIDS), and the clinical response to therapy observed when the growth of HIV is inhibited by drugs.

Perhaps the most compelling evidence for HIV as the cause of AIDS comes from studies in which people are followed over time. First, no patients develop or die from AIDS in whom the virus cannot be detected by currently available techniques. Second, the rate at which individuals progress to and die from AIDS is directly related to the amount of HIV present in the blood stream. Patients without HIV never develop AIDS; patients with low levels of virus progress slowly to AIDS; and, patients with high levels of virus progress quickly to AIDS. Other related evidence implicating HIV as the causative agent of AIDS comes from clinical trials that test drugs active against HIV. Regimens composed of drugs with potent activity against HIV prove that reducing the quantity of HIV present in blood uniformly reduces the rate at which patients progress to AIDS. These trials show that less virus leads to less HIV-related disease over time.

In addition to the nearly universal detection of HIV in patients with AIDS, meticulous studies indicate that HIV is not found outside of groups who are at risk for AIDS. Therefore, there is a very tight association between infection with HIV and both people who have AIDS and those at risk for AIDS. Many individuals found to be infected with HIV have no evidence of disease at the time of virus isolation. Detailed longitudinal studies of such people indicate that with sufficient time, most will ultimately develop AIDS. The unusual cases of long-term non-progressors (individuals with long-standing HIV infection but little clinical evidence of HIV-related disease), do not undermine HIV as the causative agent of AIDS. Studies of these individuals suggest that HIV isolated from their blood, their immune response to HIV, or both, are qualitatively different when compared with patients who have a more typical progression to AIDS. Attenuated HIV growth characteristics and an aggressive immune response to virus in patients with slow progression to disease support HIV as the causative agent of AIDS. Furthermore, laboratory work provides another form of evidence that HIV causes AIDS. Scientists showed that HIV infects and kills CD4 T-cells, the same type of lymphocyte that is depleted in people with AIDS.

Deliberately inoculating an uninfected person with HIV and observing the development of AIDS would constitute definite proof that HIV is the cause of AIDS. Although this type of inoculation will never be performed, situations that approximate direct innoculation have occurred inadvertently. Before the introduction of blood-screening procedures, direct inoculation occurred in people who unknowingly received HIV via a blood transfusion; these individuals subsequently developed AIDS and AIDS-related illnesses. Efforts to eliminate HIV from the blood supply have nearly eliminated blood transfusion as a means of transmitting HIV and with that, have essentially eliminated blood transfusion as a source of AIDS. This is further proof that HIV causes AIDS.

4. What is normal immunity?

Normal immunity is the ability of a healthy body to resist the development of disease. Resistance to disease takes place at many different levels. Any physical barrier that prevents the entry of a pathogen, a microbe, or substance that can cause disease, is in a very general way part of the immune system. Cough, intact skin, acid in the stomach, and digestive enzymes in tears are all barriers to the entry of potential pathogens.

While these physical barriers contribute to immunity, a more specific protection against pathogens occurs from a more basic defense. This defense has white blood cells as the principal component. Of the white blood cells, it is the subtype known as lymphocytes that are key to many forms of immunity and specifically those that are altered in AIDS.

There are two principal defenses mounted by the lymphocytes: the cellular immune response and the humoral immune response. T lymphocytes, a class of white blood cells, mediate the cellular immune response. When a host is invaded by a potential pathogen, T lymphocytes that recognize the pathogen are activated and attempt to eliminate the foreign agent. In HIV infection, a subset of T lymphocytes called CD4 lymphocytes are infected and killed by the HIV. It is the loss of CD4 cells that produces the immune deficiency of AIDS. In addition to lymphocytes, there are other kinds of blood cells, including monocytes, macrophages, granulocytes, and natural killer cells, that play supporting roles in the cell-mediated immune response.

The humoral immune response relies on proteins produced by B lymphocytes. B lymphocytes circulate in body fluids and become activated when they contact a pathogen. These activated cells secrete antibodies—proteins that bind directly to pathogens and facilitate their elimination from the body. Another part of the humoral immune response is complement, a set of proteins that can kill pathogens. Antibodies differ from complement in that they are directed against a specific pathogen. Complement, in contrast, may be directed against a wide range of pathogens.

Antibodies therefore are characterized by specificity whereas complement lacks specificity. Complement is not directly affected by HIV infection, but the production of antibodies is often abnormal in HIV infection.

5. What is an opportunistic infection?

Infection occurs when a microbe, such as a bacterium or virus, invades another organism, the host, and produces disease. Contact between a human and a microbe does not always produce infection; humans confront a vast array of microbes daily without being ill. Microbes fail to cause disease in humans for many reasons. Some find that the host does not offer the necessary requirements for reproduction. In addition, the lack of adequate nutrients, the presence of a harsh chemical environment, or any other impediment to the growth of the microbe render the body relatively resistant to the intruding microbe.

Examples of the effectiveness of simple physical barriers in preventing disease include bacteria that come in contact with the skin but require direct access to the blood for growth, viruses that are swallowed but inactivated by stomach acid, or fungi that require hair shafts for growth but instead find themselves on the scalp of a bald man. A microbe that successfully overcomes all of the body's physical barriers also must elude the body's immune response.

Opportunistic infections occur when normal immunity is altered. If the immune system cannot respond to a microbe that it would normally eliminate, the infection that results is termed opportunistic. It is opportunistic because it has taken advantage of decreased immunity to cause an infection that would normally not be possible.

6. How does HIV decrease immunity?

HIV preferentially infects two cell types, both part of the immune system: CD4 lymphocytes (a subset of the T lymphocytes) and macrophages.

The lymphocytes are a class of white blood cell of which there are two primary kinds: B lymphocytes and T lymphocytes. B lymphocytes secrete antibodies that are proteins directed against foreign substances including microorganisms and viruses. They are not directly infected by HIV. T lymphocytes have a wide range of functions important for activating, modulating, and effecting the immune response. The subset of T cells called the CD4 lymphocyte or T-helper cells are critically important for coordinating and carrying out much of the immune response to tumors, viruses, fungi, and other types of microorganisms. It is these types of lymphocytes that HIV selectively infects and destroys.

A second cell type infected by HIV is the macrophage. This cell participates in the immune response by interacting directly with CD4 lymphocytes.

Discoveries in the mid-1990s have shed much light on how HIV may produce loss of CD4 lymphocytes. Although many experiments are still necessary to clarify the pathogenesis of HIV-related loss of CD4 lymphocytes, broad conclusions are coming into scientific focus. A high daily production of individual HIV virons within the body is necessary for loss of CD4 cells. Scientists showed in numerous trials that administering drugs active against HIV retards and perhaps prevents the loss of CD4 cells in HIV-infected individuals. These observations indicate that the ongoing production of HIV leads to loss of CD4 lymphocytes. Scientific debate continues, however, over how viral production leads to the loss of those cells. Some proponents believe that HIV kills lymphocytes by direct infection only. Other scientists allege that because only small numbers of lymphocytes are infected with virus at any point in time, other mechanisms account for much of the loss of these cells. Many of these scientists hold that apoptosis, a process by which cells die without direct virus infection, explains the loss of CD4 cells over time. Both groups accurately cite experiments in support of their respective theories. There are insufficient data to judge the relative importance of these processes, or other processes hypothesized by scientists to account for the overall loss of CD4 cells with HIV infection. It is likely, however, that both processes contribute to the loss of lymphocytes. These two processes are probably intertwined and perhaps even dependent on each other. Whatever the specific means are by which HIV produces disease, it is now indisputable that the ongoing production of HIV is essential to the attrition of the immune system. Slowing the production of HIV, or better, erradicating the virus, will slow and perhaps prevent the deterioration of the immune system. It is not clear, however, if it will be possible to reverse any deterioration of the immune system once it occurs, even if one provides the best therapies currently available.

7. What type of virus is HIV?

HIV is a member of a group of viruses called retroviruses. As with all viruses, retroviruses are simple microscopic organisms dependent on a host for reproduction. They lack an independent metabolism and cannot grow without energy and nutrients supplied by a host cell. During infection of a host cell, retroviruses use cellular proteins to generate new genetic material and all the components from which a new virus is constructed.

Retroviruses differ from most other viruses by virtue of their reproductive strategy. In contrast with human cells as well as many other viruses that carry genetic information in the form of DNA, retroviruses carry genetic information in the form of RNA, another nucleic acid. Retroviruses convert viral RNA to DNA once the virus has infected the host cell. During infection of a host cell, retroviruses use cellular proteins to generate new genetic material and all of the components that together form the offspring virus that emerges from the infected cell. RNA is converted into DNA through a process called reverse transcription, which is the defining characteristic of all retroviruses.

Before the AIDS epidemic, retroviruses were almost unknown to physicians. The first human disease attributable to a retroviral infection was described shortly before AIDS. This disease, called adult T-cell leukemia, is an obscure cancer affecting small numbers of patients in limited geographic areas. The emergence of AIDS and adult T-cell leukemia have prompted scientists to search for retroviruses as the cause of many illnesses that are poorly understood.

8. What are retroviruses?

Retroviruses are some of the simplest viruses that exist. Their genetic information is carried in a small number of genes, almost always ten or fewer. Genes are the individual units of nucleic acid that determine hereditary characteristics. This genetic economy contrasts with the more than 500,000 genes estimated to make up the full complement of human genes. Retroviruses are roughly spherical with the outermost surface covered by a membrane (see Figure 1-1). The membrane coats a lipoprotein layer, called the envelope, which includes the viral proteins gp120 and gp41. This envelope surrounds the innermost portion of the virus called the core. The core is composed of both protein and genetic material (e.g., p24, p17), which in the case of retroviruses is carried as RNA.

The defining aspect of retroviruses is their ability to copy viral RNA into DNA by using an enzyme called reverse transcriptase (RT) (Figure 1-1). Retroviruses then integrate the viral DNA copy into the genetic material of the cells they infect using an enzyme called integrase (Figures 1-2A and 1-2B). Most viruses other than retroviruses enter a cell, reproduce, and then leave the host cell. The host cells will then either die as a result

Figure 1-1: HIV Structure. HIV has a membrane and outer lipoprotein envelope that surrounds a core containing the viral RNA genome. Reverse transcriptase (RT) is an enzyme that assists in copying of viral RNA into DNA. Glycoprotein complexes (e.g., gp41, gp120) are seen on the surface and core proteins (p17, p24) are also identified (From: *AIDS: Problems and Prospects*, by Lawrence Corey, M.D., editor. Copyright ©1993, 1992, 1991, 1990 by HP Publishing Co., New York, NY. Reprinted by permission of W.W. Norton & Company, Inc.)

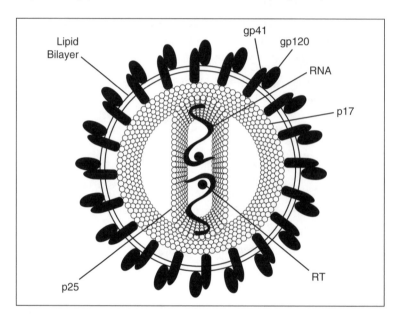

of the infection or survive with little evidence that an infection took place. In contrast, retroviruses enter a cell and remain there for the duration of the life of the cell. They copy their genetic material, RNA, into DNA which is chemically indistinguishable from the DNA found in human cells. The HIV DNA is then introduced into human DNA where the viral DNA resides for the life of the host cell. This viral genetic material serves as the blueprint for new copies of HIV.

Figures 1-2A and 1-2B: HIV Lifecycle. When HIV has fused with the cell membrane (A), the virus uncoats, bringing its core into the cytoplasm, where its reverse transcriptase (RT) initiates events that lead to production of RNA-DNA hybrids, double-stranded DNA, and finally circular but noncovalently bound cDNA copies of the viral RNA genome. The cDNA goes to the nucleus and integrates into cellular chromosomal DNA, where it may remain latent, producing little viral protein or RNA. Or, when the host cell is activated (B), viral cDNA produces mRNA, which codes for proteins necessary for virus replication and viral particles and virion RNA, which is the viral genome. The genome is packaged into infectious particles at the membrane and leaves the cell by budding, as shown, or by a poorly defined cell fusion process. (From: *AIDS: Problems and Prospects*, by Lawrence Corey, M.D., editor. Copyright ©1993, 1992, 1991, 1990 by HP Publishing Co., New York, NY. Reprinted by permission of W.W. Norton & Company, Inc.)

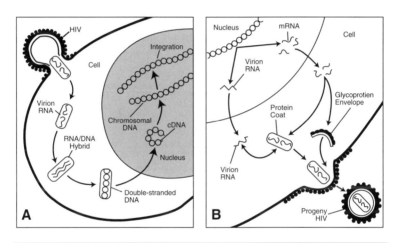

9. How did HIV originate?

Scientists can only speculate about the origins of HIV. One hypothesis is that a retrovirus related to HIV called simian immunodeficiency virus (SIV) gave rise to HIV. SIV causes an AIDS-like illness in some types of monkeys. It is possible that a retrovirus such as SIV was transmitted to humans where it did not produce disease but later evolved into the pathogen HIV. This theory is supported by the existence of HIV-2, a virus similar to

HIV that causes AIDS in western Africa. HIV-2 appears to be an intermediate form between HIV and SIV; it readily infects both humans and monkeys and causes a less severe disease than HIV or SIV in their respective natural hosts. It may be that a strain of SIV entered humans from monkeys where it then evolved into HIV-2 and finally into HIV. HIV is properly named HIV-1 to distinguish it from HIV-2, however it is almost always called simply HIV because HIV-2 is rarely found outside of western Africa.

The nature of this first entry into humans is the object of great interest and speculation. One can imagine many different ways in which humans might contact non-human primates to allow transmission of a virus. Eating, hunting, trapping, and other sorts of exposures to monkeys may facilitate transfer of a virus. It is likely that there was no one instance of a single human infection from which the current epidemic originated. Perhaps monkey retroviruses occasionally infect humans as a result of frequent contact between those two species. If that is the case, then perhaps isolated groups of people suffered from infection with HIV for decades or centuries before HIV arrived in the general population. Migration of people from rural areas to cities and the penetration of trade into previously unreached areas may have promoted dissemination of HIV outside of its original, highly circumscribed, domain. Whatever the precise historical circumstances for the first cases of human HIV infection, scientists place the origin of the current epidemic in central Africa.

Some researchers propose other explanations for the origins of the AIDS virus. A small number of scientists raised the possibility that polio vaccines produced for use in Africa were contaminated with monkey retroviruses. They proposed that the mass inoculation of this vaccine into humans introduced a virus able to reproduce in humana and then evolve into HIV. This hypothesis received little support from an investigation by an independent committee of scientists after a thorough review of the historical and scientific evidence. Likewise, there is no scientific evidence for claims that the virus was engineered by scientists and then released onto an unsuspecting public either deliberately or mistakenly.

10. Can monkey retroviruses infect humans?

Demonstrating that SIV can be transmitted from monkeys to humans may help to understand how humans were infected with HIV as well as support the hypothesis that humans were first infected with a retrovirus from monkeys. Scientists have demonstrated that SIV can infect human cells in laboratory conditions, but no experiments have examined if the virus can grow in humans. A laboratory accident in the United States indirectly tested the possibility of transmission of SIV to humans. An individual accidentally stuck with a needle containing contaminated blood from a macaque monkey infected with SIV developed antibodies against SIV proteins four months after the exposure. This raises the possibility of infection of humans by retroviruses considered unique to monkeys. In addition, a small number of animal handlers in research institutions have produced antibodies to SIV. These cases suggest that SIV can infect humans and strengthen the hypothesis that HIV evolved from a virus that first entered humans from monkeys some time in the past.

Work examining HIV-2-infected patients in western Africa identified a human infected with a strain of HIV-2 that was nearly identical to SIV. Although this patient may not have been infected with SIV, he was infected with a virus very similar to SIV. This case suggests that SIV and HIV-2 may be very close relatives. In that sense, it is plausible that all humans infected with HIV-2 are actually infected with a form of SIV.

—CHAPTER TWO—

The Manifestations of HIV Infection

11. What is the definition of AIDS?

On January 1, 1993 the Centers for Disease Control (CDC) expanded the definition of AIDS to include an extensive list of diseases reflecting advanced HIV infection and CD4 lymphocyte numbers indicative of significantly compromised immunity. This definition revised two earlier versions also offered by the CDC.

The first definition, put in place in 1981 before the discovery of HIV, was purely clinical and was limited by the unavailability of laboratory indicators of HIV infection. This original definition was revised in 1987 to expand the number of opportunistic infections and malignancies indicative of AIDS and to include the results of newly available laboratory tests.

Physicians recognized that some conditions occuring frequently in AIDS patients were not included in earlier definitions of AIDS. The 1993 definition therefore incorporated new clinical manifestations of severe HIV-related disease. This new definition also incorporated low CD4 cell numbers or percentage of CD4-to-total lymphocytes as diagnostic of AIDS. This modification of the definition of AIDS reflected the close relationship between susceptibility to opportunistic disease and low CD4 cell numbers. AIDS is now defined for individuals aged 13 years or older as documented HIV infection and any one of the following:

A. Fewer than 200 CD4 cells per microliter of blood
B. Less than 14% of all lymphocytes are CD4 cells

C. At least one of the following medical conditions:
1. Candidiasis of bronchi, trachea, or lungs
2. Candidiasis, esophageal
3. Invasive cervical cancer
4. Coccidioidomycosis, disseminated or extrapulmonary
5. Cryptococcoses, extrapulmonary
6. Cryptosporidiosis, chronic intestinal (more than one month's duration)
7. Cytomegalovirus disease (other than liver, spleen or nodes)
8. Cytomegalovirus retinitis (with loss of vision)
9. Encephalopathy, HIV-related
10. Herpes simplex: chronic ulcer(s) (more than one month's duration); or bronchitis, pneumonitis, or esophagitis
11. Histoplasmosis, disseminated or extrapulmonary
12. Isosporiasis, chronic intestinal (more than one month's duration)
13. Kaposi's sarcoma
14. Lymphoma, Burkitt's (or equivalent term)
15. Lymphoma, immunoblastic (or equivalent term)
16. Lymphoma, primary, of brain
17. *Mycobacterium avium* complex or *M kansasii*, disseminated or extrapulmonary
18. *Mycobacterium tuberculosis*, any site (pulmonary or extrapulmonary)
19. *Mycobacterium*, other species or unidentified species, disseminated or extrapulmonary
20. *Pneumocystis carinii* pneumonia
21. Pneumonia, recurrent
22. Progressive multifocal leukoencephalopathy
23. *Salmonella* septicemia, recurrent
24. Toxoplasmosis of the brain
25. Wasting syndrome due to HIV

The case definitions for children and adults are the same with the exception that lymphoid interstitial pneumonitis (LIP) and recurrent, serious bacterial infection are added to the case definition for children. Each of these conditions will be discussed.

12. What is the natural history of infection with HIV?

HIV infection causes clinical disease and immunological abnormalities by gradually destroying the immune system. Because of the progressive nature of the illness, the stages of disease are somewhat arbitrarily chosen although some clear distinctions exist.

For example, a patient recently infected with HIV is very different from a patient with long-standing HIV infection. Although both patients suffer from HIV infection, patients with early infection usually have no or only minor symptoms, while those further along in the course of HIV infection can have profound immune deficiency and are at risk for AIDS, the terminal phase of HIV infection. These two stages of disease are easily differentiated, but intermediate stages are much less so. It is this blurring of the borders between stages that makes tracking subtle distinctions in HIV-related illness difficult.

The full spectrum of HIV-related illness has become apparent because laboratory testing can now detect the presence of HIV before illness develops. No diagnostic tests were available in the early years of the epidemic. As a consequence, physicians relied on a description of the clinical illness to both diagnose and count AIDS cases. The development of diagnostic testing has helped to understand the earliest stages of HIV-related illness. These stages include many conditions not meeting the definition of AIDS although they are caused by HIV infection.

Physicians now understand that immediately after infection with HIV, a series of events are set in motion. These events can lead to AIDS. Patients first experience an acute illness known either as primary HIV infection or acute retroviral illness within days or weeks after infection. Symptoms accompanying primary infection are usually transient and are the first clinical evidence that a person is infected with HIV.

Some weeks after a primary illness, most people become asymptomatic. Once asymptomatic, they have little to no outward evidence of their disease in many cases for ten years or more although immunological abnormalities are detectable using laboratory techniques. These abnormalities become increasingly apparent as the CD4 cell count progressively decreases. If HIV infection was not diagnosed during primary infection, and it usually is not, then these people may be unaware of their infection until developing an AIDS-defining illness. If they continue to engage in the behaviors that led to HIV infection, then they may infect others.

After several years of carrying HIV and, in many cases, unwittingly passing the virus on to others, the infected person may become aware of abnormalities for the first time. Some patients will experience persistent generalized lymphadenopathy, or enlarged lymph glands throughout the body; others may develop constitutional symptoms such as fever, weight loss, diarrhea, and lethargy. These symptoms were previously referred to as ARC or AIDS-Related Complex and are now called HIV-symptomatic disease. Both of these conditions were at first thought to be subcategories of HIV infection with important prognostic information, and their presence was incorrectly thought to indicate an increased risk of progressing to AIDS.

Physicians now pay less attention to these manifestations of HIV infection for prognostic purposes and focus instead on laboratory assessments. The levels of HIV in blood and circulating CD4 lymphocyte levels have much more prognostic information for HIV-infected persons than clinical findings such as the state of lymph nodes or constitutional symptoms including fever or weight loss.

As the CD4 count decreases from its normal level of approximately 1,000 cells/μL to levels below 500, people become at risk for opportunistic infections. Although the risk is low around 500 cells, it increases substantially at counts below 200.

Most patients will experience symptoms of some kind below 200 cells, whether as a result of opportunistic infection or constitutional symptoms. At counts below 100, patients are at great risk for opportunistic infections and at counts below 50, the survival of most people is limited to months.

13. What is the incubation period for AIDS?

The incubation period for AIDS is the time that elapses between HIV infection and the development of an AIDS-defining condition. This time is measured as the *median* time or interval during which one-half of all patients will develop AIDS. One-half of all patients will therefore not develop AIDS during the median incubation interval.

The median time between infection with HIV and the development of an AIDS-defining condition is about ten years. A large study of homosexual men from San Francisco initially helped define the incubation period of patients infected with HIV. Of the 288 men in this study, 33% developed AIDS 4.5 years after infection. Mathematical modeling of this group predicted a median of 10 years for the development of AIDS.

Another study of 75 homosexual men with persistent generalized lymphadenopathy found that 48% of these patients progressed to AIDS in 9 years, a figure consistent with other studies. Subsequent evidence suggests that rates of progression to AIDS for heterosexuals and intravenous drug users are similar to rates for male homosexuals.

A lengthening median incubation period to longer than 10 years would indicate a slowing progression to AIDS. There are several reasons why the progression of disease may be slowing and the median incubation period may be increasing. Significant recent improvements in antiretroviral therapy and the prevention of opportunistic infections are profoundly influencing the rate of HIV disease progression. The extent of the delay in disease progression, however, is not yet fully known. Other reasons why disease progression may be slowing include modification of behaviors to decrease the chances of encountering unidentified factors that might accelerate the activity of HIV, improved medical care, and perhaps the evolution of HIV to less pathogenic strains. The median time to progression to AIDS is based on studies completed during the early years of the epidemic and may not apply to those infected now, many of whom may benefit from new therapies.

The effect of therapeutic advances on slowing of HIV disease progression was first noted by scientists examining the incidence of AIDS cases in the United States after introduction of zidovudine (ZDV) in 1987. Scientists found a clear decrease in the expected number of HIV-infected persons progressing to AIDS. The greatest decline was in HIV-infected white male homosexuals who received treatment for HIV infection more frequently than other groups. This decrease in new AIDS cases was attributed primarily to treatment of HIV and to the initiation of widespread preventive therapy of *Pneumocystis carinii* pneumonia, the most common opportunistic infection. Additional therapeutic advances such as use of protease inhibitors are likely to further slow the progression of HIV infection and reduce the incidence of AIDS beyond reductions already observed with ZDV.

14. How long will persons remain asymptomatic after infection?

Patients become symptomatic at various stages of HIV infection. Symptoms associated with primary infection occur at the outset of infection and usually dissipate rapidly. Patients may develop additional symptoms such as diarrhea or enlarged lymph nodes months to years following infection. These HIV-related symptoms by themselves so not meet the case definition of AIDS. Persons vary greatly in the time it takes to develop AIDS. Some individuals progress to AIDS in well under two years after HIV infection while the longest time between infection and the first appearance of AIDS is not well defined. There are numerous people infected with HIV since the early 1980s without clinically apparent disease.

Physicians believe, however, that most HIV-infected individuals who do not receive effective therapy will develop AIDS if their life is not cut short by some other unrelated event. The median time from HIV infection until development of an AIDS-defining opportunistic infection is about 10 years and most people remain asymptomatic for prolonged periods before developing AIDS. Many HIV-infected persons, however, have clinical manifestations associated with HIV infection before meeting the clinical or laboratory criteria that define AIDS.

Laboratory indices predict the development of AIDS very accurately. The most useful laboratory indicator of disease progression is the level of HIV present in the bloodstream. Clinical studies using sensitive techniques such as the polymerase chain reaction assay (PCR) or the branched DNA assay (bDNA) established the relationship between rates of progression of HIV disease and the level of HIV in blood. Scientists now know that a single determination of HIV levels is highly prognostic in estimating risk of disease progression in patients. In all cases, low levels of HIV are indicative of a better prognosis, either for risk of developing an AIDS-related condition or death, than higher levels of HIV.

The factors that influence the level of HIV present in a given individual are obscure at this time. In general, patients are evenly distributed around a median value with some having very low levels and others having very high levels. It is likely that many factors contribute to the level of HIV achieved in patients, and thus affect the period of time between infection and onset of symptomatic HIV disease. For example, the strain (type) of HIV with which infection occurs, the amount of virus with which the person is infected, the pre-existing state of the immune system, and the ability to mount an adequate immune response all probably interact to set a baseline level from which HIV tends to grow in any given patient. At this time, there is no way to estimate the level of HIV in the blood of a patient without directly measuring that level. Studies have made it clear that the primary goal of therapy must be to reduce the level of HIV present in blood if one hopes to retard or prevent disease progression. Drugs that accomplish this goal are increasingly available with an expanding array of antiretroviral agents that have been developed since the start of the AIDS epidemic.

15. What are the different stages of HIV infection?

The presence of selected opportunistic illnesses and laboratory criteria define AIDS. However, the majority of HIV-infected persons do not have AIDS by the CDC definition because they have yet to develop an AIDS-defining opportunistic illness and have a CD4 count greater than 200 cells/μL.

A staging system has been developed by the CDC to classify persons with HIV infection at all points between initial infection and AIDS based on clinical findings and CD4 cell numbers. This classification allows physicians to better communicate with each other and with their patients. It allows the use of a common terminology to describe research results, and to develop prognostic information helpful to those with HIV infection. In the absence of such a system, the description of patients is imprecise and communication of clinical information is made difficult.

The CDC classification system for HIV infection was revised in January 1993 and replaces the classification system introduced in 1986 (Figure 2-1). It uses an assessment of a person's clinical condition as well as incorporates the results of CD4 cell counts. As mentioned in the previous discussion, in many respects the utility of a CD4 cell-based scheme is very limited. It tells little about the future, but does provide information on the current state of the immune system.

The classification system revised in 1993 readily categorizes all HIV-infected persons. Many patients do not progress through each of the stages of HIV disease; some patients may move from

Figure 2-1: The CDC January 1993 HIV classification

CD4 T-cell categories	Clinical Categories		
	A Asymptomatic, acute (primary) HIV or PGL*	B Symptomatic, not (A) or (C) conditions	C AIDS-indicator conditions
1. ≥ 500/µL	A1	B1	C1
2. 200-499/µL	A2	B2	C2
3. < 200/µL	A3	B3	C3

PGL=persistent generalized lymphadenopathy

an early to a late stage without passing through any of the intermediate stages in either system. Other classification schemes have been proposed, but at this time there is no uniform clinical staging system used by all physicians.

The CDC used a different system to classify HIV infection before the revised definition of AIDS and HIV classification introduced in 1993. This system is found throughout the medical literature on HIV before 1993 and is included here for reference purposes (Figure 2-2). The classification scheme was not devised to provide prognostic information or to define the severity of HIV illness. The scheme was, instead, intended to allow better health care planning, improve public health control strategies, and to provide more comprehensive epidemiological data and optimal patient care among those not meeting the CDC definition of AIDS. The scheme was hierarchical in the sense that persons could only be classified into more advanced groups as their symptoms and signs progressed.

These classification schemes provide very limited prognostic information. There is little relationship between the stage a patient has reached and time to death. Much more prognostic

Figure 2-2: HIV classification system before 1993.

Group I	Acute infection
Group II	Asymptomatic infection
Group III	Persistent Generalized Lymphadenopathy (PGL)
Group IV	Other Disease
Subgroup A	Constitutional Disease (previously ARC and including symptoms of persistent fever, weight loss, or diarrhea and not explained by a concurrent condition other than HIV infection)
Subgroup B	Neurological Disease (dementia, myelopathy or peripheral neuropathy)
Subgroup C	Infectious Diseases
Subgroup C-1	Specific infectious diseases listed in the CDC definition of AIDS
Subgroup C-2	Any 1 of 6 other infections: oral hairy leukoplakia; herpes zoster involving multiple nerve distributions; recurrent salmonella bacteremia; nocardiosis; tuberculosis; or oral candidiasis
Subgroup D	Specific cancers listed in the CDC definition of AIDS
Subgroup E	Other disease related to HIV infection but neither infectious nor neoplastic. Also included are patients with symptoms that are not otherwise classifiable.

information comes from the level of HIV present in the bloodstream than from the CDC classification scheme. As additional experience accumulates with assay systems that measure the level of HIV in the blood, such as the PCR or bDNA assays, it is probable that these techniques will supplant the current CDC system of HIV classification.

16. What is "acute HIV infection?

Acute or primary HIV infection occurs when HIV first enters the body, encounters the immune system, and begins production of new HIV, called viral replication. Scientists have found that the virus grows rapidly in the days after first infection; viral proteins are often detectable in serum and cerebrospinal fluid, the liquid that bathes the brain and spinal cord, often before the antibodies they elicit are made.

As seroconversion—the appearance of antibodies directed against HIV proteins—occurs, the levels of virus and p24, a readily measured protein component of HIV, decrease and virus becomes difficult to isolate. The decrease in virus reflects the immune response of the body. Antibodies scavenge viral proteins and inactivate newly produced virus; cell-mediated immunity also reduces the level of virus in the body. While the level of HIV in some body fluids decreases, it is the inability of the immune response to eliminate virus that leads to chronic infection.

Most infected persons develop antibodies weeks to a few months after HIV infection, but some research studies using sophisticated techniques have identified evidence of HIV infection up to 18 months before seroconversion is detectable by standard tests. These results are subject to interpretation, but if true, probably apply to only a very small percentage of all persons who are infected with HIV. Nonetheless, there may be some individuals infected with HIV who do not develop antibody evidence of HIV infection until months after their initial contact with the virus. Although these individuals are infected with HIV, the inability to elicit a rapid antibody response and its meaning for infectiousness is under study.

17. What are the symptoms associated with acute HIV infection?

Many individuals develop symptoms associated with primary HIV infection within two to four weeks after infection with the virus. These symptoms include an acute transient illness with fever, muscle aches, headaches, rash, and sore throat. Many persons also experience a sense of fatigue and malaise, and lymph nodes often enlarge around the time of seroconversion, the point where antibodies against HIV are first produced. Oral, anal, and penile ulcers develop in many cases. Some persons report gastrointestinal symptoms including nausea, vomiting, and diarrhea. Early HIV infection may quickly affect the nervous system and cause brain, spinal cord, and peripheral nerve damage.

Not all persons have symptoms with primary HIV infection. Those who are symptomatic usually have symptoms limited to less than two weeks, although a few persons experience lingering problems for months. Prospective studies following individuals at risk for HIV infection found that from 50% to 70% of people report the symptoms of primary HIV infection at the time of seroconversion. Other studies asked already infected persons about symptoms suggestive of HIV infection experienced in the past. They found that over 90% recollected an illness consistent with primary HIV infection. Preliminary information suggests that people who have a protracted or symptomatic illness associated with primary HIV infection may progress to AIDS more rapidly than those who do not have symptoms. In addition, preliminary studies suggest that antiretroviral therapy administered during primary HIV infection may improve at least the early subsequent clinical course of the disease.

18. What are some of the early symptoms following acute HIV infection?

After the symptoms associated with primary HIV infection disappear, most people will not experience any evidence of their HIV disease until several years elapse. It is in this period of relative health that individuals, called carriers, often transmit HIV to other people. The healthy carrier is often unaware of his or her infection and may take no additional precautions to prevent transmission of HIV.

The first symptoms that people experience usually several years after primary infection were once termed "ARC" or AIDS-related complex, a name now superseded by the term HIV-symptomatic disease. These symptoms include weight loss and wasting, enlarged lymph nodes, fever without an identifiable source, diarrhea, and lethargy. Patients also experience fungal infections such as oral thrush, and herpes zoster, a viral condition causing disseminated vesicles on the skin. Although each of these infections is treatable, they can cause much discomfort.

Another early symptom of HIV infection is enlarged lymph nodes, alternatively known as persistent generalized lymphadenopathy (PGL). The importance of this condition is similar to that of ARC. Originally thought to be a unique aspect of HIV infection with a distinct natural history and rate of progression to AIDS, it is now viewed as an early manifestation of HIV infection, and the clinical course of those with it is not different from those HIV-infected persons without it.

19. What are the symptoms of AIDS?

AIDS is the final stage of HIV infection and is characterized by profound immunodeficiency. This stage of HIV infection occurs when the immune system is exhausted and incapable of producing sufficient CD4 lymphocytes to defend the body against most pathogens normally controlled by those cells when present in adequate numbers.

AIDS by itself is not a condition characterized by specific symptoms. Instead, the symptoms experienced by patients with AIDS are determined by the opportunistic illness that occurs as a result of the immunodeficiency induced by HIV. Symptoms will therefore differ from person to person depending on the opportunistic illness or illnesses that afflict any one patient. HIV infection can cause some clinical manifestations by itself without an accompanying opportunistic illness. For example, HIV causes neurologic abnormalities as a result of direct infection of the brain and spinal cord, but opportunistic infections cause the majority of the medical problems experienced by patients with AIDS. Virtually all parts of the body can be affected by one or another opportunistic infection. The most common symptoms reflect the most frequently occurring opportunistic infections. The vast majority of patients will experience symptoms related to the lungs such as coughing or shortness of breath. Many others have headache, seizures, and loss of normal thought processes as a result of brain infections. Another common symptom is diarrhea from a number of causes, and many patients have painful or debilitating abnormalities of the skin and eyes from viral infections. The various manifestations of AIDS and opportunistic infections will be discussed.

—CHAPTER THREE—

Opportunistic Infections

20. What role do opportunistic infections play in AIDS?

Opportunistic infections cause most of the morbidity and mortality in AIDS. During autopsy, close to 100% of AIDS patients have at least one opportunistic infection. In the absence of therapy directed against HIV, treatment and prevention of opportunistic infections hold the greatest promise for improvements in the prognosis of those with AIDS. It may be possible that patients could continue to be infected with HIV, perhaps indefinitely, if no opportunistic illnesses occur.

Physicians formerly relied primarily on the presence of opportunistic infections to diagnose AIDS. AIDS-defining opportunistic infections were used because they are convenient indicators of the severity of immunodeficiency, are easily observable, and do not require frequent laboratory monitoring as is the case with CD4 cells. Although tracking opportunistic infections was very useful in the early years of the AIDS epidemic, other tests now surpass their utility in finding cases of HIV infection and in staging the illness. These tests quantitate the number of individual viruses present in blood. They more accurately predict the course of HIV-related illness than opportunistic infections.

Opportunistic infections, however, continue to play a major role in the diagnosis of AIDS. In addition, the presence of any AIDS-defining opportunistic infection in a person who is HIV infected require reporting to local and national health authorities for epidemiological purposes.

The common opportunistic infections can be organized by the organs they affect.

Lungs: This is the most commonly involved organ system in AIDS because it represents a portal of entry for inhaled microorganisms. The lungs are the principal target for *Pneumocystis carinii* and are also commonly the site for cytomegalovirus, *Cryptococcus neoformans*, and a variety of typical and atypical tuberculous bacteria (e.g., *Mycobacterium*). It is not unusual for several of these organisms to infect a person with AIDS simultaneously. During the autopsy, many patients are found to have died of respiratory failure caused by an opportunistic infection affecting the lung.

Skin: This is the preferred site for the cancer Kaposi's sarcoma. Herpes simplex and varicella-zoster viruses can cause painful, deep, and destructive ulcers in many different locations on the skin. Molluscum contagiosum, a disfiguring viral disease, sometimes affects the genitals and the anal region with venereal warts.

Gastrointestinal: The gastrointestinal tract can be affected anywhere between the lips and the anus. Commonly found microorganisms include the herpes simplex virus that can cause an inflammation of the esophagus called esophagitis and *Candida albicans*, a fungus that causes both oral thrush and esophagitis. Other microorganisms cause intestinal disturbances resulting in debilitating diarrhea and malabsorption of food. These microorganisms include *Cryptosporidium*, cytomegalovirus, *Isospora belli*, and *Mycobacterium avium-intracellulare*. Oral hairy leukoplakia, a white plaque-like lesion of the tongue and mouth associated with Epstein-Barr virus, is an important early symptom in persons with HIV infection.

Lymph nodes: These can undergo changes from direct infection by organisms such as *Cryptococcus* or tuberculous bacteria, infiltration by tumor cells of Kaposi's sarcoma, or as the result of infection in the part of the body that is drained by that node.

Eyes: A sizable proportion of persons with AIDS have cytomegalovirus retinitis, an inflammatory condition of the retina (the sensory portion of the eye). Cytomegalovirus retinitis commonly results in blindness.

Brain: A majority of persons with AIDS have dramatic changes in the diverse functions of the brain sometime during the course of their disease. Opportunistic infections causing brain disease in persons with AIDS include toxoplasmosis from the protozoan *Toxoplasma gondii*, meningitis from *Cryptococcus neoformans*, and progressive multifocal leukoencephalopathy, a viral illness that kills selected cells in the brain.

Many persons who are not infected with HIV may develop disease from infection with one of these microorganisms. In all cases, the disease by itself does not warrant the diagnosis of AIDS unless also accompanied by HIV infection.

21. What is oral hairy leukoplakia?

Oral hairy leukoplakia (OHL) is a condition found frequently in people with HIV infection, and its presence alone is not sufficient for a diagnosis of AIDS. OHL consists of white plaques that often coat the tongue. Although the cause of the lesion is uncertain, electron microscopic examination has found evidence of Epstein-Barr virus in the lesions. OHL is usually asymptomatic and rarely requires therapy, but treatment with acyclovir or ganciclovir, a drug related to acyclovir, is reported to exert some beneficial effect.

22. What is Pneumocystis carinii?

Pneumocystis carinii is a microorganism that causes a disproportionately large percentage of all opportunistic infections in AIDS. Its precise biological classification remains unclear. Most experts categorize it as a fungus, while others consider it a protozoan. In the early years of the epidemic, *Pneumocystis carinii* pneumonia (PCP) was the first AIDS-defining opportunistic infection in approximately three of every five AIDS patients. With the advent of preventative therapies, the incidence of PCP has decreased. However, PCP remains the most common opportunistic disease affecting patients with AIDS and represents a major cause of morbidity and mortality.

As is the case with other opportunistic infections, the incidence of PCP is closely linked to the state of the immune system. The majority of PCP cases occur at CD4 levels that are less than 100; cases rarely occur at CD4 cell counts greater than 200. Patients with PCP often have the following symptoms: fever, progressive shortness of breath, and a dry cough. Medical evaluation typically reveals a chest x-ray pattern that is often sufficiently characteristic to allow the initiation of therapy without additional diagnostic tests. In those cases that require additional investigation, the diagnosis is made either by examining sputum for presence of the organism or by collecting material directly from the lungs via a procedure called bronchoscopy.

The rapid diagnosis of PCP is essential to a satisfactory outcome. Patients with delayed therapy may die from the pneumonia. In the early days of the AIDS epidemic, when the diagnosis of PCP was not made as quickly as it is today, patients rarely recovered from PCP. Because of the high incidence of PCP, physicians now diagnose the illness in its early stages and initiate effective antibiotic therapy before the pneumonia progresses to an advanced stage. Despite the use of effective therapy, patients may never eradicate the organism from their lungs. Therefore, after an episode of PCP or at CD4 cell counts less than 200, the CDC recommends that all HIV-infected patients receive antibiotic prophylaxis to prevent infection or recurrence of clinical disease. Numerous studies document the effectiveness of prophylactic regimens in the prevention of PCP.

23. What is Kaposi's sarcoma?

Kaposi's sarcoma (KS), a rare cancer that affected mainly older men of Mediterranean descent before the AIDS epidemic, is now found in many patients with AIDS. In patients without AIDS, KS grows slowly and is confined to the skin and lymph nodes. In AIDS-related cases, the disease appears as painless reddish-blue to brown skin lesions, either soft or firm, most often on the legs. Lesions may spread with time to other portions of the skin, primarily on the head, neck, and mouth. Later, lymph nodes may enlarge, signaling involvement of the lymphatic system. It may further spread into the internal organs, especially the lungs and gastrointestinal tract.

KS, the most common cancer in AIDS, appeared in 15% of all US AIDS patients from the onset of the AIDS epidemic in 1981 through 1991. The disease has an incidence of about 45% in homosexual men but only about 3% in individuals with intravenous drug use as their risk factor for infection. These discordant rates of disease incidence supported a transmissible agent as the source of KS.

For many years during the early stages of the AIDS epidemic, the cause of KS was unkown. In 1995 researchers in New York City found that a virus belonging to the herpes family was frequently associated with the tumor. Subsequent work established the link of this virus, now know as either Kaposi's sarcoma herpes virus or as human herpes virus 8 (HHV-8), to the disease.

Epidemiological observations find that the median time after infection with HHV-8 before the development of KS is about 33 months. Further studies are underway to determine the prevalence of HHV-8 infections in the general population, although small studies indicate that it is low. Early work suggests that the virus may be aquired through sexual contact. While additional research remains to be completed to understand how the virus interacts with the cells it infects and how to intervene successfully to stop the growth of the tumor, it appears that HHV-8 at least contributes to and may cause KS.

There are no known means to prevent KS other than maintaining an intact immune system. Because the presence of HHV-8 appears to be important, if not essential, in developing KS, avoiding infection with this virus may lower the likelihood of developing KS. One can only speculate that, if sexual contact is the primary route of spread of HHV-8, reducing the number of sexual contacts may lower the likelihood of coming in contact with HHV-8.

KS is not curable with currently available therapies and no therapies are known that are active specifically against HHV-8. The treatment of KS uses chemotherapy that often includes alpha interferon, a product that the body generates in response to viral infections. Radiation therapy improves inaccessible lesions inside the body and lesions not responding to drug treatment. KS is usually not life threatening and most affected persons die of other opportunistic infections. Early studies found that AIDS patients who had KS but no other opportunistic infection, survived a median of 30 months and patients with both PCP and KS lived a median of 14 months. Improved antiretroviral therapy should extend these survival rates. Limited information also suggests that the use of protease inhibitors in the treatment of HIV infection can improve, but not cure, KS.

24. What is toxoplasmosis?

Toxoplasmosis is the disease resulting from infection with *Toxoplasma gondii*. This organism commonly infects adults throughout the world and typically resides in the body without evidence of clinical illness. The ingestion of food containing *Toxoplasma* cysts are the principal route of transmission of this particular protozoan which persists latently inside of the cells that it infects. Individuals with normally functioning immune systems rarely develop disease from *Toxoplasma*, however, patients with HIV infection are prone to reactivation of the organism and subsequent illness.

Reports state that up to 40% of those with AIDS and anti-bodies to *T. gondii* develop toxoplasmosis in the brain, with a one year incidence of about 25% in patients with CD4 counts less than 100/μL. This infection becomes clinically apparent usually well after the patient has experienced other opportunistic illnesses, but in a small percentage of patients, toxoplasmosis can be the first opportunistic infection. Most patients with central nervous system toxoplasmosis develop headache, confusion, fever and, often, seizures. Some of these patients will have neurologic deficits leading to weakness, poor coordination, and confusion. Most patients will respond to standard therapy in two weeks, but to maintain the initial response, patients require longterm therapy because relapses following the cessation of therapy are common. Patients who have prior exposure to *T. gondii* as indicated by the presence of antibodies directed against *Toxoplasma*, and who have CD4 counts less than 100/μL, should receive prophylactic therapy.

25. What is Mycobacterium avium complex (MAC)?

MAC consists of several species of bacteria (e.g., *M. avium* and *M. intracellulare*) that rarely cause disease in normal hosts, but that cause one of the most common systemic bacterial infections in patients with AIDS. It is the third most frequent opportunistic disease affecting patients with AIDS, and is estimated to affect up to 40% of patients within two years of diagnosis of AIDS.

MAC usually occurs late in the course of HIV infection and especially with CD4 counts less than 100 cells/uL. The blood is the most frequent site of infection, and organ involvement, especially the liver, spleen and bone marrow, is also common. Fever, night sweats, fatigue, abdominal pain, and weight loss—while seen with other conditions—are features of disseminated MAC disease and are associated with shortened survival. Combination antimicrobial therapy can reduce the morbidity associated with MAC, and recent studies have shown that prophylactic regimes in those with CD4 counts less than 100/µL result in beneficial clinical effects.

26. What is candidiasis?

Candida albicans causes candidiasis, a fungal infection that occurs frequently in patients with HIV infection. It is found most commonly in the mouth, where it is called thrush, and in the esophagus. It appears as a white exudate coating the affected tissues but is often painless when present in small amounts. Severe *Candida* infections of the back of the mouth and esophagus are often associated with pain when swallowing. Localized *Candida* also can occur elsewhere in the body, although the gastrointestinal tract is, by far, the most frequently affected site. Systemic disseminated *Candida* infection is rare in patients with HIV infection.

Localized *Candida* infection is a treatable condition. Numerous anti-fungal therapies exist which are either applied topically to the affected oral tissue or, for cases resistant to topical therapy, ingested. Because *Candida* is found throughout the environment and reinfection readily takes place, many patients will require long-term suppressive therapy to prevent its recurrence.

27. What are other fungal infections that affect AIDS patients?

Cryptococcus neoformans, *Histoplasma capsulatum*, and *Coccidioides immitis* are all fungi that cause disease in AIDS patients. AIDS surveillance data collected by the CDC document that *Cryptococcus* causes disease in at least 5% of AIDS patients in the United States. This fungus is found throughout the world and is highly associated with pigeon droppings. The fungus first enters the lungs, and can pass to the central nervous system, where it often causes meningitis. The meningitis can be treated with several different antifungals including amphotericin B, fluconazole, and itraconazole, but chronic therapy is necessary to suppress recurrence of disease. Untreated cryptococcal meningitis usually ends in death.

Histoplasmosis, caused by *Histoplasma capsulatum*, is found principally in the Ohio and Mississippi River valleys in the United States and in parts of Africa and Latin America, with occasional cases in Europe and other areas scattered around the world. Histoplasmosis usually causes pulmonary disease, the lungs being the site of entry into the body. Patients also develop a myriad of clinical problems caused by dissemination of the organism throughout the body, including arthritis, cardiac problems, and liver and skin infections.

Coccidioidomycosis also disseminates widely throughout the body, although it has a predilection for the brain where it causes severe meningitis. As with *Cryptococcus*, similar therapeutic approaches for both histoplasmosis and coccidioidomycosis apply; patients require intense treatment with an antifungal drug and then maintenance therapy for the duration of the patient's life.

28. What is cryptosporidiosis?

Cryptosporidiosis, caused by the protozoan *Cryptosporidium*, is a watery diarrhea found in many with AIDS. Patients experience severe abdominal pain, malaise, and weight loss due to malabsorption. Some patients may lose over 20 liters of fluid per day through diarrhea which leads to severe dehydration. Because the organism is shed into the feces, it is transmissible to others through contaminated water and close contact. Limited evidence also supports transmission of the organism through contaminated food, sexual contact, and perhaps coughing.

Household disinfectants, freezing, and heating all kill the organism. Although the organism can be killed outside the body, no highly successful treatment is known for the clinical condition.

Antibiotics have not been found useful; other therapeutic approaches using less traditional treatments including bovine colostrum, bovine immunoglobulins, and other protein products remain unproved.

29. What is isosporiasis?

Isosporiasis, caused by the microorganism *Isospora belli*, is another cause of diarrhea in AIDS patients. Although the mode of transmission is undetermined, the organism is found throughout the world and is especially prevalent in the tropics. American AIDS patients suffer from diarrhea caused by *Isospora* in only about one in 200 cases, but in Haiti more than one in 10 patients will develop isosporiasis. Individuals with adequately functioning immune systems who are infected with *Isospora* have symptoms that resolve spontaneously. AIDS patients, however, suffer from a prolonged illness that will, despite therapy, relapse. Patients report watery diarrhea, weight loss, and pain in the abdomen. Although many patients benefit from extended therapy with various antibiotics, withdrawal of therapy often leads to a recurrence of the disease.

30. What is zoster?

Zoster, commonly called shingles, is a painful infection of the skin caused by the varicella zoster virus (VZV). VZV causes chicken pox, a common childhood illness that rapidly resolves. After chicken pox, VZV persists as a chronic infection and remains within the nerves of the face, trunk, and pelvis. In normal hosts, the infection occasionally reactivates and causes lesions reminiscent of chicken pox over certain areas of the skin. This reactivation, more commonly known as shingles, is painful but usually short lived.

Zoster in AIDS patients is typically neither limited to a particular area of the skin, nor limited in duration. Pain in the area frequently accompanies the lesions. VZV typically affects large areas of skin in immunosuppressed individuals and can involve other organs of the body not usually affected in immunocompetent people. Some patients also experience involvement of the central nervous system with signs of encephalitis (infection of the brain) including confusion, headache, loss of coordination, and seizures. The infection can be controlled and sometimes reversed by treating the patient with the antiviral compound acyclovir. High daily doses are required to exert an effect that may be accompanied by side effects or even eventual resistance of the virus to the drug.

31. What is herpes simplex?

There are two different viruses that carry the name herpes simplex: herpes simplex type 1 (HSV-1) and herpes simplex type 2 (HSV-2). These viruses can cause clinical syndromes that are nearly identical, and the viruses themselves are distinguishable only by laboratory techniques. As is the case with other members of the herpes family of viruses including the Epstein-Barr virus, cytomegalovirus, varicella-zoster virus, and human herpes virus 6, infection is lifelong and reactivation can be frequent and unpredictable.

Both HSV-1 and HSV-2 persist in the sensory nerves of the skin. Reactivation of the infection often results in herpes, a condition of painful vesicles on skin supplied by the involved sensory nerve. Although HSV-1 usually persists in the nerves of the face and HSV-2 most frequently persists in the nerves of the lower trunk and genitals, either virus can be found in either location. Herpes is a common sexually transmitted disease in individuals with normal immune systems. In this population, scattered lesions in the affected area appear after a first infection or following reactivations of the initial infection. The lesions are usually painful and are highly infectious; however, with time, they recede and leave no evidence of their presence.

AIDS patients can suffer profound symptoms with reactivation of herpes virus infection. The virus often creates large ulcers in mucocutaneous areas such as at the edge and inside of the mouth, near the genitals, and around the anus. These ulcers are contagious and extremely painful. They rarely improve spontaneously because a normal immune system is necessary for resolution of symptoms. Instead, AIDS patients often have a lingering or expanding lesion that may become infected with bacteria, thus necessitating antibiotic therapy. These lesions often respond to treatment with the antiherpetic drug acyclovir. Unfortunately however, the required prolonged treatment and inability to eradicate the virus from the body can generate strains resistant to acyclovir. Other compounds that are active against HSV exist, although their side effects are more severe and, in some cases, must be administered via intravenous infusion.

32. What is cytomegalovirus?

Cytomegalovirus (CMV) is a member of the herpesvirus family. Although it is occasionally a pathogen in people with apparently normal immune systems, cytomegalovirus often causes a common and debilitating infection in patients with advanced AIDS. Many individuals are infected with the virus in early life-primarily through close contact with others. Clinical disease in these circumstances is infrequent and usually not severe. Once infected, the body harbors the virus indefinitely. In settings of immune suppression, either as a result of a malignancy, medical treatment, or AIDS, the virus can reactivate and cause disease.

CMV disease appears in the latest stages of AIDS when CD4 cell levels are well below 50/µL. The most common manifestation of CMV is retinitis, an infection of the nerve layer in the back of the eye. This condition afflicts about one-third of AIDS patients and, if left untreated, usually ends in blindness.

Other clinical conditions include CMV pneumonia, colitis (infection of the colon), encephalitis, and occasionally adrenalitis (infection of the adrenal glands). Colitis is associated with diarrhea and gastrointestinal pain, encephalitis leads to headache and other neurologic abnormalities, and adrenalitis can lead to low blood pressure.

CMV is readily diagnosed by detection in a culture or by microscopic visualization in affected tissue. Three drugs, foscarnet, ganciclovir, and cefpodovir, have demonstrated efficacy in the treatment of retinitis and can prevent or delay the onset of blindness. Each of these drugs requires intravenous administration for an indefinite period of time and is associated with significant and sometimes limiting toxicities, or side effects. Oral ganciclovir used prophylactically reduces but does not eliminate the risk of CMV disease in infected individuals. Attempting to avoid the virus if one is not already infected may be best done by avoiding transfusion with blood products from a CMV-infected donor. The prevalence of CMV infection in AIDS patients, however, is very high—as many as 90% of AIDS patients have evidence of CMV infection at autopsy.

33. What is progressive multifocal leukoencephalopathy?

Progressive multifocal leukoencephalopathy, or PML, is a viral illness found in 4% to 7% of those with AIDS. Patients with PML suffer neurological symptoms such as progressive limb weakness, incoordination, decreasing visual acuity, and ultimately profound dementia. The clinical condition is caused by infection with JC virus, named in recognition of the patient from whom it was first isolated. Growth of the virus destroys cells necessary for the proper functioning of the brain.

Up to 60% of adults indefinitely harbor the JC virus in an inactive form within their body after infection during childhood. The reappearance of the latent virus takes place in the late stages of AIDS when profound immune deficiency occurs. Before

AIDS, cases of PML were rare and these were reported in patients whose immunosuppression was caused by conditions other than AIDS. There is no specific therapy for PML other than reducing the underlying immune suppression which allows it to occur.

34. What are Non-Hodgkin's lymphomas?

Lymphomas are a form of cancer of the lymphocytes. The lymphomas that occur in AIDS are usually malignancies of B cells, the type of lymphocyte responsible for secreting antibodies. A related lymphoma, called Hodgkin's disease, is distinguishable from lymphomas by its pathologic appearance, clinical course, and response to therapy. Up to 10% of AIDS patients may develop a Non-Hodgkin's lymphoma, usually during the later stage of HIV disease. With the advent of retroviral therapy, malignancies that were not seen in the early stages of the epidemic have become more common. The appearance of these lymphomas does not indicate that the natural history of AIDS is changing. Rather, it implies that patients now live long enough to experience consequences of immune deficiency that appear much later in the disease.

Therapy for these malignancies is rarely curative. Because treatment regimens usually include drugs that damage the immune system, AIDS patients must receive less chemotherapy than if they had normal immune systems. Some of the best chemotherapy regimens lead to a response in about 50% of patients and give a median survival of a little over one year.

AIDS patients also experience other lymphomas of the brain that are rarely diagnosed in patients with normal immune systems. These malignancies respond poorly to radiation therapy directed at the brain—currently the best treatment available.

35. What is cervical dysplasia?

A very high rate of abnormal Pap smears has been found in HIV-infected women. The Pap smear is a routine technique used to detect cancer of the cervix, the structure at the back of the vagina. The most common abnormality is dysplasia, the abnormal growth of cells on the surface of the cervix. Cervical dysplasia increases in incidence as the CD4 cell count falls below 400 cells. Although dysplasia is not cancer, it is viewed as a precancerous lesion in normal women. Studies are now underway to determine the rate at which this lesion progresses to cervical cancer in women with HIV infection.

A virus called human papillomavirus (HPV) is strongly associated with cervical dysplasia. This virus is often spread sexually and may be the causative agent for the cervical abnormalities. It also infects men in whom it can cause venereal warts. Surgery is used to treat cervical disease. The abnormal tissue is readily accessible through the vagina where it can be excised, or cut out, under direct visualization. Studies are in progress to further understand how the disease begins and to identify simple procedures that will prevent its occurrence.

36. What causes the wasting syndrome in patients with HIV infection?

Wasting, or the progressive decrease in body cell mass manifested as weight loss, is a common problem during infection with HIV. Body cell mass is lost when caloric intake, the energy ingested, is less than the energy used. Insufficient calories to meet energy use can occur when a loss of appetite or food malabsorption prevents the uptake of enough calories to match the rate of their use by the body. Disordered metabolic processes that do not transport calories into cells also contribute to this mismatch. The rate of metabolism of the body determines the use of calories. An increased metabolic rate is the usual reason for increasing caloric consumption above normal. Metabolism is usually increased through exercise, and healthy individuals who exercise compensate for increased energy demands by eating more food. HIV infection, on the other hand, also can increase metabolism and result in a hypermetabolic state. Patients with hypermetabolic states, not induced by exercise but instead by severe HIV infections or burns, cannot adapt by simply eating more food.

The body has an intricate system for controlling the disposition of calories. Cytokines, a class of molecules that mediate immune function, also influence how calories are used. It may be that because many cytokines are active during HIV infection, patients with HIV often become hypermetabolic. Experiments demonstrate that even patients without clinical signs of HIV infection have an increased metabolism. These patients usually do not lose weight early in infection, but instead minimize energy expenditure by reducing activity while experiencing fatigue and listlessness. These symptoms are a physiologic adaptation to minimize demand for calories.

All AIDS patients ultimately experience wasting to some degree. As illness progresses, the wasting caused by the hypermetabolism of infection may be compounded by malabsorption, diarrhea, and other gastrointestinal problems. Nausea and anorexia reduce appetite, fever and infection increase the metabolic rate, intestinal disease generates malabsorption, and an active immune response interferes with the proper handling of energy.

Progressive wasting in AIDS patients is particularly severe in Africa. Wasting is sometimes the most prominent form of HIV infection in Africa, and the local population calls it "slim disease." Severity of wasting in Africa is a function of the lack of access to medical care and nutrition and not a manifestation of HIV infection peculiar to Africans.

37. Can HIV-infected persons reduce the risk of acquiring opportunistic infections?

Microorganisms responsible for most opportunistic infections are present throughout the environment, although there is a geographical restriction to some pathogens. There are at least five ways to reduce the risk of acquiring an opportunistic infection.

First, and most important, patients should attempt to maintain the integrity of the immune system. A relatively intact immune system will minimize the risk of infection after an encounter with an opportunistic pathogen. The best way to retard the decline in immune function during HIV infection is through the use of appropriate antiretroviral therapy. Several studies indicate that delaying deterioration of the immune system through the use of antiretroviral agents reduces the risk for opportunistic disease. An emerging consensus derived from many different clinical trials using diverse therapeutic agents holds that immune deterioration can be limited most successfully by using regimens that reduce the amount of virus in the blood to the lowest possible levels.

Second, patients can take a drug that reduces the likelihood of developing clinical disease or relapse after an encounter with a potential pathogen. This approach is called prophylaxis. The likelihood of developing opportunistic infections increases at CD4 cell counts below 200. Therefore, the National Institute of Allergy and Infectious Diseases recommends measuring CD4 cell levels every three months once the counts fall to about 300. Testing this frequently should detect the point at which patients will begin to benefit from prophylaxis against *Pneumocystis carinii* pneumonia, the most common opportunistic infection and one associated with substantial morbidity and mortality. *Pneumocystis carinii* is one of the organisms for which prophylactic regimens are most clearly defined, and therapeutic regimens usually consist of antibiotics containing sulfamethoxazole and trimethoprim. Physicians also use antibiotics, either a macrolide or rifabutin, to prevent infection with *Mycobacterium avium* complex (MAC). Physicians frequently initiate MAC prophylaxis at CD4 cell counts below 100. The risk of CMV disease may also be reduced by providing oral ganciclovir to patients with less than 50 CD4 cells. Evidence also supports the efficacy of antimicrobial therapy to prevent toxoplasmosis in selected patients at risk for the disease.

The third form of risk reduction prevents contact with the offending pathogen. In most cases, this is an almost impossible feat. HIV-infected persons, however, can take some precautions, but there is little to no formal evidence that they are effective. Some physicians recommend that patients avoid eating uncooked fish or meat. These foods can contain protozoa and bacteria that can produce devastating infections in immunocompromised hosts. Because cat feces are frequently contaminated with *Toxoplasma gondii* cysts, persons without previous exposure and pre-existing immunity to this microorganism should minimize contact with litter boxes. *Cryptosporidium* is not a common pathogen in the United States, but it is very prevalent in some developing countries. Boiling water before drinking should eliminate the risk of consuming viable organisms. *Isospora belli*, a parasite of the gastrointestinal tract, is found throughout the Caribbean and requires prolonged treatment once contracted. Again, water that is boiled before drinking should eliminate the possibility of infection with this organism. Those with immune suppression should consider the relative risks of infection with these pathogens before traveling to the areas where they are found.

The fourth measure that may be beneficial in warding off an opportunistic infection includes vaccination when possible. Many physicians recommend vaccination with the pneumococcal vaccine, the hepatitis B vaccine, the influenza vaccine, and the *Hemophilus influenzae* vaccine when appropriate in HIV infection. Most patients with early HIV infection will develop immunity against these common pathogens from vaccination and may derive benefit from its use.

A fifth approach that is used to avoid significant morbidity from opportunistic infections relies on aggressively treating the disease as soon as it becomes apparent. High quality medical care, with appropriately directed physical and laboratory examinations, can detect many abnormalities in their earliest stages before they become more difficult to treat. Laboratory screening of high risk populations for syphilis, searching for enlarged lymph nodes, examining the eyes, and routinely observing the skin, are all ways to detect illnesses that commonly occur in these areas, therefore allowing the initiation of therapy at the earliest possible stage. In practice, elements of all of these forms of avoiding opportunistic infections should be used by patients with HIV infection who are significantly immuno-compromised.

38. Can a person have an opportunistic infection and a low CD4 cell count without actually being HIV infected?

Patients with opportunistic infections and low CD4 counts but no evidence of HIV infection were first reported in 1992. Except for the absence of HIV infection, these patients did meet the case definition of AIDS. Fearing a possible new epidemic, public health officials raised the possibility of a transmissible agent, other than HIV, that was able to cause this AIDS-like illness. However, there is no virological or epidemiological evidence that this illness is caused by an unusual strain of HIV, or any other transmissible agent.

Researchers attempting to collect similar cases have not established the cause of the deficient immunity in these patients. Some scientists hypothesize that the low CD4 levels may be an unusual consequence of the infecting opportunistic pathogen. Others have suggested that a very small number of patients may normally have persistently low CD4 cell counts. There is no evidence that this syndrome, recognized in fewer than several hundred patients worldwide, is a new form of AIDS.

39. What symptoms of AIDS are not caused by opportunistic infections?

The most prominent symptoms unrelated to opportunistic infections are neurologic. Over 15% of adults with AIDS, but up to 50% of children with AIDS, have progressive deterioration of cognition or thinking. This condition, termed AIDS Dementia Complex (ADC) in adults and HIV-1-associated progressive encephalopathy in children, often entails the slowing of mental processes, difficulty in concentration, apathy, personality changes, memory defects, and alterations in the level of consciousness. This dementia, or intellectual deterioration, is not attributable to opportunistic infections of the brain or depression, both capable of causing altered mental function. Many persons with ADC also have difficulties with unsteady gait, leg weakness, and a loss of coordination. These additional problems stem from degeneration of the spinal cord, termed myelopathy.

Symptoms of ADC are thought to result from direct infection of the brain with HIV. Scientists know HIV can infect brain and spinal cord tissue in the early stages of infection. In addition to brain and spinal cord, HIV also affects peripheral nerves. These structures carry impulses to and from the spinal cord and brain. Impairment of peripheral nerves responsible for sensation causes numbness and pain, most prominently in the feet. HIV affects the motor neurons, the nerves that carry impulses to muscles. Damaged motor neurons weaken muscles, a problem compounded by muscle weakness resulting as a side effect of HIV treatments.

The first definition of AIDS did not recognize the neurological abnormalities common in AIDS patients. After the recognition of ADC, the definition of AIDS was revised in 1987 to include HIV-related neurological disease that results from direct HIV infection without secondary opportunistic infections or cancers. Although many patients suffer from neurological problems during HIV infection, many do not. Why the nervous system in some patients is adversely affected and why it is not in others is incompletely understood.

40. Does HIV infection differ in women and men?

Early in the epidemic, the number of men with HIV infection in developed countries vastly exceeded the number of women with HIV infection. The relative lack of women with HIV infection led to an underrepresentation of women in clinical studies. This underrepresentation contributed to a less complete understanding of HIV infection in women than in men.

In the United States, women infected with HIV acquire the virus more from the use of intravenously injected drugs than from sexual exposures. This is usually true in other industrialized countries but less so in developing countries where sexual contact remains the major source of infection. The progression of HIV disease does not appear to differ in infected women who used injecting drugs compared with infected women who do not.

In addition, clinical studies indicate that, when treated with similar therapies, women as a group have rates of progression to an AIDS-defining illness similar to those seen in male study populations. While some studies have found HIV-infected women who actively use intravenous drugs have poorer outcomes than men in similar circumstances, differences in medical care may account for this disparity. Investigations examining whether pregnancy accelerates HIV-disease progression have also found inconsistent results. It is clear, however, that HIV infection during pregnancy transmits HIV to the child in one in three instances if antiretroviral treatment is not administered.

Women do have some manifestations of HIV infection that are different from those of men. These different manifestation include vaginal candidiasis, (an infection with the fungus *Candida*); genital papillomavirus infections; and pelvic inflammatory disease, a painful condition of the genital tract that may be caused by a number of different microorganisms. The incidence of some malignancies differs between women and men. Kaposi's sarcoma, a cancer affecting skin and lymph nodes, is relatively infrequent in HIV-infected women; however, abnormalities of the cervical tissue, including a greatly increased incidence of precancerous lesions, are greatly increased in HIV-infected women when compared with uninfected women.

There is little information concerning the differences between women and men on the effects of various therapies directed at HIV infection, although there seems little reason to believe that the benefits and side effects of existing drugs used to treat HIV infection in women should be very different from those found in men. Only long-term studies of both existing and investigational agents that include adequate numbers of women will rectify this lack of information.

41. How does HIV affect children?

HIV infection, as in adults, causes immune suppression in children that culminates in opportunistic infections. Although most children infected with HIV appear normal at birth, within 24 months about 80% will begin to show some symptoms of disease. Predicting the risk for opportunistic disease is more difficult in children than in adults. In children the CD4 lymphocyte level has less value as a prognostic indicator than it does in adults; a child may become ill with opportunistic infections at a higher CD4 cell count than would an adult.

Some AIDS-related conditions are more prominent in children than in adults. Infected children experience problems with bacterial infections affecting the ears, bones, brain, and joints more frequently than adults. Brain disease caused by direct infection of the brain by HIV (termed HIV-1-associated progressive encephalopathy) causes intellectual deterioration and developmental regression in both cognitive and motor function in children. The encephalopathy may also cause progressive weakness affecting the legs first and then the arms and trunk.

Developmental delay is found in up to 90% of children with HIV infection. In addition, lymphoid interstitial pneumonitis (LIP), a form of inflammation of the lung associated with progressively worsening lung function, is found in up to 40% of children. HIV-infected children otherwise have many of the same problems that plague adults with AIDS. As is often the case, however, the manifestations and treatment of a given infection in children are not identical with those in adults.

Reports of children born with physical abnormalities as a result of *in utero* infection lack confirmation. Early in the AIDS epidemic 20 children were described with growth failure, a small head circumference and an unusual appearance consisting of a prominent forehead, a short nose with a flattened bridge, a prominent upper lip, and atypical eyes. In contrast with this report, most observers find that, whether or not the child is infected, the vast majority of children born to HIV-infected mothers are clinically normal at birth.

There are unique issues associated with the development of drugs used in the treatment of HIV-infected children. The testing of investigational drugs for treatment of HIV and opportunistic infections in children is usually conducted after the evaluation of these compounds in adults. Studies of new therapies for AIDS, as well as other illnesses, are traditionally conducted first in adults and then in children. This conservative approach minimizes the risk of exposing children to new drugs before the side effect profile in adults is understood. The lack of effective therapies for HIV has reduced the delay between studying drugs in children and adults; although, in most cases, children are not given access to new HIV therapies as quickly as adults are.

—CHAPTER FOUR—

Transmission of HIV

42. Who gets AIDS?

In the United States, AIDS cases have been reported from every state with the highest rates in New York, California, Florida, Texas, and New Jersey; and the lowest rates in Montana, Wyoming, and the Dakotas. As of June, 1996, 548,102 AIDS cases were reported to the CDC. Of these cases, 540,806 were either adults or adolescents and 7,296 were children 13 years of age or younger. The breakdown of AIDS cases in the United States by type of exposure, age, sex, and race/ethnicity is displayed in Figures 4-1 and 4-2.

43. What are the principal routes of HIV transmission?

HIV is transmitted through three routes: sexual exposure, contact with blood contaminated with HIV, and transmission from a mother to a child through pregnancy and birth. Examination of the various groups with HIV infection shows that the vast majority of people are infected through sexual contact of one form or another. Statistics reveal that over one-half of all cumulative AIDS cases in the United States in 1996 were in homosexual and bisexual men. This statistic is deceptive, however, because it does not show the trend of infection in different groups. In the earliest stages of the AIDS epidemic in both the United States and in Europe, homosexual and bisexual men accounted for upwards of 90% of all cases. Intravenous drug users were a small minority of all cases limited to only a few geographic areas, and heterosexual cases were distinctly unusual outside of Africa.

Figure 4-1: Who gets AIDS? AIDS cases by type of exposure, reported through June 1996, United States (548,102 total cases).

Adults and Adolescents (540,806 cases)

51%   Men who have sex with other men
25%   Heterosexual intravenous drug users
 7%   Men who have sex with other men and use intravenous drugs
 8%   Heterosexual contact:
      Sex with HIV-infected person, unspecified risk group (46%)
      Sex with IV drug user (45% of heterosexual cases)
      Sex with bisexual male (5%)
      Sex with transfusion recipient with HIV infection (2%)
      Sex with person with hemophilia (2%)
 7%   Other or undetermined*
 1%   Recipients of infected blood transfusion, blood components or tissue
 1%   Hemophilia/coagulation disorders

Children and infants (7,296 cases)

90%   Born to mother with HIV or at risk for it
 5%   Recipient of infected blood product or tissue
 3%   Hemophilia/coagulation disorders
 1%   Other or undetermined**

*   *Other* refers to 24 health care workers who developed AIDS after occupational exposure (e.g., needlestick injury or mucocutaneous exposure to blood) to HIV-infected blood; 39 persons who acquired HIV infection perinatally but who were diagnosed with AIDS after age 13; and one person who developed AIDS after intentional self-inoculation.

Undetermined includes persons possibly infected through heterosexual contact with a partner at high risk for HIV infection but whose infection status was unknown; persons who chose not to disclose high risk information; and persons with possible occupational exposure to infected blood or other body fluids. This group also includes persons unavailable because of death, refusal to be interviewed, or inability to be located

**   Includes two children who were exposed to HIV-infected blood in a household setting.

Centers for Disease Control and Prevention, Atlanta, Georgia, 1996.

Table 4-2: AIDS cases by age, sex, race/ethnicity, reported through June 1996, United States.

MALES

Age at diagnosis	White Not Hispanic No. (%)	Black Not Hispanic No. (%)	Hispanic No. (%)	Asian/ Pacific Islander No. (%)	American Indian/ Alaska Native No. (%)	Total* No. (%)
< 5	443 (0)	1763 (1)	665 (1)	15 (0)	9 (1)	2,899 (1)
5-12	303 (0)	322 (0)	217 (0)	8 (0)	1 (0)	853 (0)
13-19	726 (0)	560 (0)	327 (0)	19 (1)	14 (1)	1,647 (0)
20-24	6,541 (3)	5,216 (4)	3,119 (4)	113 (3)	50 (4)	15,061 (3)
25-29	32,478 (14)	19,120 (13)	12,349 (15)	438 (13)	243 (20)	64,715 (14)
30-34	55,851 (24)	31,102 (22)	19,276 (24)	741 (22)	327 (27)	107,431 (23)
35-39	53,259 (22)	32,876 (23)	17,778 (22)	736 (22)	260 (21)	105,062 (23)
40-44	38,581 (16)	24,637 (17)	12,121 (15)	602 (18)	167 (14)	76,218 (16)
45-49	22,940 (10)	13,285 (9)	6,628 (8)	349 (10)	73 (6)	43,335 (9)
50-54	12,267 (5)	7,027 (5)	3,460 (4)	182 (5)	29 (2)	22,997 (5)
55-59	6,765 (3)	3,900 (3)	1,979 (2)	112 (3)	19 (2)	12,804 (3)
60-64	3,884 (2)	2,094 (1)	1,078 (1)	46 (1)	12 (1)	7,123 (2)
65+	3,198 (1)	1,685 (1)	811 (1)	50 (1)	8 (1)	5,759 (1)

Male Subtotals:

237,236(100) 143,587(100) 79,808(100) 3,411(100) 1,212(100) 465,904 (100)

FEMALES

Age at diagnosis	White Not Hispanic No. (%)	Black Not Hispanic No. (%)	Hispanic No. (%)	Asian/ Pacific Islander No. (%)	American Indian/ Alaska Native No. (%)	Total* No. (%)
< 5	434 (2)	1,776 (4)	648 (4)	11 (3)	12 (5)	2,888 (4)
5-12	134 (1)	340 (1)	173 (1)	6 (1)	— —	656 (1)
13-19	169 (1)	605 (1)	145 (1)	6 (1)	1 (0)	927 (1)
20-24	1,171 (6)	2,666 (6)	1,048 (6)	24 (6)	22 (10)	4,936 (6)
25-29	3,316 (17)	6,996 (15)	2,913 (17)	45 (11)	39 (17)	13,316 (16)
30-34	4,461 (23)	10,441 (23)	4,028 (24)	82 (20)	51 (22)	19,092 (23)
35-39	3,685 (19)	9,956 (22)	3,363 (20)	75 (18)	43 (19)	17,156 (21)
40-44	2,324 (12)	6,399 (14)	2,079 (12)	59 (14)	21 (9)	10,892 (13)
45-49	1,200 (6)	2,864 (6)	1,070 (6)	39 (9)	20 (9)	5,199 (6)
50-54	676 (4)	1,489 (3)	602 (4)	21 (5)	8 (4)	2,799 (3)
55-59	502 (3)	845 (2)	373 (2)	11 (3)	5 (2)	1,738 (2)
60-64	359 (2)	536 (1)	188 (1)	17 (4)	3 (1)	1,103 (1)
65+	794 (4)	504 (1)	175 (1)	19 (5)	2 (1)	1,496 (2)

Female Subtotals:

19,225(100) 45,417(100) 16,805(100) 415(100) 227(100) 82,198 (100)

TOTALS, Male and Female:

256,461 189,004 96,613 3,826 1,439 548,102 (100)

* Includes 650 males and 109 females whose race/ethnicity is unknown.

Centers for Disease Control and Prevention, Atlanta, Georgia, 1996.

Africa did, however, serve as an example of what could happen. The epidemic in Africa, more widespread than in developed countries, was almost exclusively in heterosexuals. Over the first decade of the AIDS epidemic in developed countries, the virus has moved across groups gaining access to new populations through individuals who overlapped two different groups. HIV appeared first in the male homosexual population in the developed world, and until 1987, AIDS was thought to be a disease exclusively of homosexuals. Bisexual men and male homosexual drug users formed a ready bridge from the first affected population to others who were not gay. The female partners of bisexual men encountered HIV by sexual relations with their counterparts who acquired HIV from exposures to infected men. Because of the common practice of sharing needles after injecting drugs into the bloodstream, infected drug users passed HIV on to those with whom they shared needles and syringes, or to sexual partners. Drug-using homosexuals also introduced the virus into the drug-using population, both male and female. A large portion of female prostitutes also inject drugs. They, by virtue of their frequent contact with heterosexual men, introduced HIV into male populations that neither injected drugs nor who were homosexuals.

HIV-infected blood served to transmit the virus to groups other than drug users. Before 1985 an individual who might have been at risk for HIV infection could donate blood for medical purposes. Recipients of either a blood transfusion or any type of different human blood products before 1985 were at risk for infection with HIV regardless of drug use or sex practices.

Children, as well as fetuses, comprise the final group at risk for HIV infection. Children born to women infected with HIV continue to be a source of new infections. Although not reflected in the reported numbers of AIDS cases, uninfected children also suffer from AIDS by outliving their infected parents who die of AIDS.

The mode of HIV transmission may influence the likelihood that an exposed individual will become infected. Health care workers exposed to an HIV-contaminated syringe have an estimated seroconversion rate of less than 0.4%. Infants born to untreated HIV-infected women have an approximate 25% risk of infection. These differences probably reflect the amount of virus in an individual exposure. In addition, the risk of a single unprotected sexual exposure to HIV is most likely low. This risk is influenced by the type of intercourse as well as nutritional, medical, and genetic factors. For example, the presence of genital ulcers or other breaks in the skin or mucous membranes increases the susceptibility to infection with HIV. On the other hand, a small proportion of people appear to be relatively resistant to HIV infection by virtue of the presence of a mutated protein on cells of their immune system.

44. Which body fluids contain HIV?

HIV is present in many body fluids. Despite its presence throughout the body, the principal forms of transmission are limited to direct exposure to contaminated blood, sexual contact with exposure to either male or female secretions, and exchange of blood from mother to child during pregnancy or shortly thereafter. Organs and sperm from HIV-infected donors also are efficient ways of transmitting HIV. Prospective donors of these tissues are now screened routinely for presence of HIV and contaminated material is discarded. Scientists have created a list of other body fluids that contain HIV, but in virtually every case other than the primary routes, HIV is recovered only with difficulty or is not thought to be a route of transmission of the virus. Figure 4-3 lists different body fluids and their different methods for HIV transmission.

Figure 4-3: Methods of HIV transmission for various body fluids.

Body site or product	HIV present	Transmission
Blood	yes	Sharing needles, contaminated blood transfusion, blood product, maternal-fetal transfer
Breast milk	yes	Maternal-child transfer
Cerebrospinal fluid	yes	Health worker exposure
Feces	yes	Implicated in a case of exposure to bloody feces
Saliva	yes	Suspected in a case of exposure to bloody saliva
Semen	yes	Sexual intercourse, insemination
Skin	no	
Tears	yes	Unproved as a route of transmission
Human tissue	yes	Organ transplantation
Urine	yes	Unproved as a route of transmission
Vaginal/cervical secretions	yes	Genital to oral contact and genital to genital contact

45. How is HIV spread through sexual intercourse? Are women more susceptible to HIV infection from intercourse than men?

Transmission of HIV from men to women and from women to men is well documented, although the exact risk of transmission per single exposure is unknown. The transmission from men to women is fairly well understood. Semen from an infected man contains HIV that is most likely associated with infected lymphocytes that are also present in semen. HIV introduced into the vagina must make its way into the blood stream to initiate viral reproduction. Small breaks in the lining of the vagina are the presumed entry to the bloodstream.

Some studies indicate that women may be more susceptible to infection than men after a single exposure to HIV. This difference may be attributable to the greater number of potential entry sites in the vagina than on the surface of the penis and because the vagina is exposed to a greater volume of infectious material than is the penis.

Although female-to-male transmission clearly occurs, the means of transmission of HIV from women to men is less clear. Studies conducted in Africa demonstrated a clear relationship between HIV infection in men and the presence of genital ulcers. Physicians hypothesize that genital ulcers in men serve the same function as breaks in the lining of the vagina by providing the virus a portal of entry to the bloodstream. A genital ulcer is not required, however, for HIV transmission to take place.

Other factors undoubtedly play a role in how readily the virus is exchanged between individuals during heterosexual genital intercourse. The presence of the menses, simultaneous infection with other organisms, cutaneous conditions, prior exposure to chemical irritants that disrupt the skin, and other conditions may all play a role in the transmission of HIV. In most of these cases, definitive answers that accurately assess the relative contribution of each factor to the risk of transmission will be difficult to achieve.

46. When does semen first contain HIV?

A small study examined semen at various intervals after primary infection. In each of the three patients, one or another laboratory technique found evidence of HIV in semen, regardless of the use of zidovudine, during the four weeks following the first clinical evidence of infection. The earliest point that a newly infected individual can transmit HIV to another person via semen is not known. However, any HIV-infected man should be considered infectious and capable of transmitting HIV at any time during the course of his infection. The widespread presence of HIV throughout the body during primary infection and the evidence of HIV in semen within weeks of infection suggests that individuals recently infected with HIV are probably infectious in the earliest stages of HIV infection.

The presence of virus in semen presents grave risks to women who are uninfected but wish to become impregnated by an infected man. Very limited research has demonstrated the feasibility of inactivating virus in infected semen, artificially inseminating a woman, and avoiding infection in both the woman and the child. Doctors have induced only a tiny number of pregnancies through this procedure; it is consequently only a research procedure with very limited availability.

Artificial insemination by a donor other than the infected sex partner does not completely avoid the risk of infection with HIV. There are several well-documented cases of HIV transmission via artificial insemination with the semen of a man not initially recognized as being infected. Recommendations for artificial insemination now require HIV screening for all sperm donors. Sperm collected from HIV-antibody negative donors is stored frozen until demonstration of a second negative antibody test after at least two to four months. There is then only a vanishingly small chance that the donated sperm contains HIV after two negative tests separated by this period.

47. What is the risk to heterosexuals of acquiring HIV infection?

Researchers attempted to define the percentage of heterosexual adults at risk for HIV infection by conducting a large survey during 1992 of more than 10,000 heterosexual individuals in the United States. The study, designed to reflect the general heterosexual population, included people aged 18 to 75 and collected data on both sexual habits and on condom use. Participants were then classified into groups that were judged to be either at risk or not at risk for HIV infection. The groups at risk included those who reported multiple sex partners, had sex with a partner from a risk group, had received a transfusion, reported intravenous drug use, or who had any combination of these behaviors.

Respondents who reported at least two different sex partners in the last twelve months were considered to have multiple sex partners. Those who admitted to injecting cocaine, heroin, speed, or steroids in the preceding five years were considered drug users. Sex partners from a risk group were those known to be infected with HIV, had used intravenous drugs in the preceding five years, were not monogamous, had received a transfusion, or were a hemophiliac. Participants who received a blood transfusion between 1978 and 1985 and had not been tested for HIV were also judged to be at risk for HIV infection both for themselves and for their partners.

The results demonstrated that at least 15% of the general heterosexual population in the United States is at risk for HIV infection through either a behavior or through an exposure to blood. The results are tabulated in Figure 4-4, where the percentage for each group within the general heterosexual population is shown.

Respondents were taken at their word and when they claimed to not know or not recall, they were not assigned to a risk group. If one assumed that respondents who could not recall or did not know the answer to a question were attempting to conceal information that would have revealed a risk factor, then the estimated percentage of heterosexuals from the general population with some kind of a risk factor for HIV infection increased dramatically to 39.8%. These high rates of risk behaviors pose grave dangers for the general heterosexual population. More recent studies have corroborated the conclusion that a significant proportion of heterosexuals are at high risk for HIV infection.

Figure 4-4: Risk groups for HIV infection within the heterosexual population, 18 to 75 years of age, 1992, United States.

Risk Group	Percentage
Multiple partners*	7.0
Partner at risk	3.2
Transfusion recipient	2.3
Multiple partners and risky partner	1.7
Multiple partner and transfusion recipient	0.0
Risky partner and transfusion recipient	0.2
All others**	0.7
No risk	84.9

* Within the past 12 months
** IV drug users, IV drug users and other combinations, hemophiliacs and combinations of three or more different risks.

Although it is impossible to assign an accurate risk of HIV infection to an individual, the uninterrupted practice of risk behaviors will allow HIV to continue to spread across the heterosexual population.

48. What is the risk of HIV infection per episode of vaginal intercourse with an infected partner?

This risk is difficult to measure precisely, but some reasonable estimates can be made based on data collected in a large study completed in Europe. In this study, 304 HIV-negative subjects and their partners were evaluated. This includied 196 women and 108 men, whose only risk factor for HIV infection was a sexual relationship with an HIV-infected person. These couples were followed for an average of 20 months during which time they were tested for evidence of HIV infection. Although about 40% of all couples ceased sexual relations usually due to the death or illness of the infected partner, 256 couples continued to have sexual relations for at least three months while in the study.

About 48% of the study participants used condoms consistent-ly, while the remaining couples used them inconsistently or not at all. Among the couples using condoms, none of the subjects became infected with HIV. The couples engaged in a minimum estimate of 15,000 episodes of intercourse. Of the group in which condoms were used less reliably, about 4.8 seroconversions occurred per 100 person years of study.

Of the couples who used condoms inconsistently, the estimated rate of transmission was about 1 per 1000 episodes of intercourse. The risk quintupled if the partner had advanced AIDS, and decreased to about 0.7 per 1000 episodes of intercourse if the partner was asymptomatic. Of note in this study was the lack of a clear difference in the rate of transmission from men to women compared with rate of transmission from women to men, although this may be a function of the small number of individuals who seroconverted. Other studies indicate that women are infected by men at about twice the rate per episode of intercourse than are men by women.

Other findings in this study included genital ulcers as a risk factor for infection. The presence of genital ulcers increased the risk of infection about five-fold above those without an ulcer. After 24 months, the cumulative rate of seroconversion in this group was estimated to be about 40%, a very high number. Un-protected anal intercourse appeared to confer a small additional risk of infection above those who engaged in anal intercourse with a condom, but the very small number of couples who parti-cipated in unprotected anal intercourse may lead to an inaccurate estimate of the risk of this particular sex act. The cumulative rate of seroconversion in couples engaging in unprotected anal intercourse after 24 months of follow-up was about 28%.

Withdrawal before ejaculation conferred a significant protective effect over those who did not withdraw. Of those couples in whom withdrawal before ejaculation was carried out in at least 50% of intercourse episodes, there was a five-fold reduction in risk compared with those couples who did not withdraw before ejaculation.

In addition, 39 couples had unprotected oral sex despite consistently using a condom during vaginal intercourse. No seroconversions were found in this group. One cannot conclude that there is no risk of HIV infection from unprotected oral sex. However, it is therefore estimated that no more than 4.7 individuals would be infected during 100 person years of this sex act as carried out in the study population. Once again, the relatively modest number of subjects who fell into this group limited the ability to make precise estimates of the rate of transmission by oral sex.

The results of this study apply to individuals who continue sexual relations with the same person over an extended period of time. Individuals who engage in any of the sex acts described with multiple sex partners may have very different risks for infection. In particular, work from Southeast Asia found that the risk of infection per sexual act could be as high as 1 in 20 to 30 episodes when the studied population engage routinely in sex with prostitutes. In either case, numerous lines of evidence now support the use of condoms as a way of preventing transmission during sexual relations.

49. What are the risks for wider spread of HIV in the heterosexual population?

Africa is a model for the spread of HIV within the heterosexual population in the absence of public health measures. The very high prevalence of HIV in heterosexuals of either sex in central Africa indicates that HIV can spread through a large heterosexual population, although it is highly unlikely that a similarly high prevalence will soon develop in industrialized countries. Awareness of the disease, better access to medical care, and its confinement to circumscribed populations should keep the prevalence of infection much lower than in Africa.

Researchers can only attempt to predict the rate at which HIV will spread in the North American and European heterosexual population. Surveys investigating heterosexual sex and rate of partner change can estimate the time necessary to double the number of HIV-infected people in the population. Scientists have estimated that if the sexually active heterosexual population averaged a sex partner change every one to two years, the prevalence of the virus in the general heterosexual population would double approximately every two years. The actual rate of doubling in heterosexuals is lower than this and lower than in male homosexuals in the early years of the epidemic. Some reasons that may account for this difference include a less efficient transmission of the virus among heterosexuals, a slower average rate of partner turnover, and a lower rate of anal sex compared with male homosexuals. There may be groups, especially sexually active young people, who change partners near or above this rate. These groups of people are at especially high risk to spread the virus from person to person.

50. How is HIV transmitted by homosexual intercourse?

Male homosexuals engage in a variety of sex practices, several of which result in exposure to semen, blood, and feces. These bodily fluids may be introduced to another partner through the mouth, genitals, or rectum. It is difficult to assess the relative risk of each sex practice for HIV transmission, but contact with blood and semen are widely held to be the principal routes by which the virus is transmitted.

Rectal intercourse appears to be the primary means by which HIV is transmitted in homosexuals. Rectal intercourse often leads to breaks in the lining of the rectum. These breaks in the rectal lining make it easier for HIV to enter into the bloodstream. Some laboratory studies suggest that cells that line the rectum may also become directly infected with the virus, although these studies were performed with cells adapted to grow under laboratory conditions and may not reflect what actually occurs within the body.

The risk of infection per individual exposure is difficult to calculate. Surveys of the gay population indicate that an insertive partner seems to have a lower chance of becoming infected than the receptive partner when the opposite individual is infected. Both of these activities, when performed without any physical barriers to HIV, however, must be considered as high risk for transmission of the virus.

51. Are lesbians at risk for HIV infection?

HIV infection is less common among lesbians than among heterosexual women, almost certainly because of their limited exposure to body fluids that carry HIV. Two case reports in which women became infected after engaging in oral-genital and oral-anal sex indicate that transmission via these routes is possible. But HIV infection in women who engage in sex solely with other women is highly unusual, after women who also use intravenous drugs are excluded. It seems that lesbians are as susceptible as any other person to infection with HIV, and have no difference in risk for aquiring HIV when well-recognized risk behaviors (e.g., injecting drug use) are practiced. However, it is important to note that oral-genital and oral-anal sex are behaviors in which the risk of HIV transmission is real, but incompletely defined for both men and women, whether heterosexual or homosexual.

52. Why do homosexual men form a large percentage of all AIDS cases?

The homosexual connection with HIV infection has been both distorted and misinterpreted, particularly in the early years of the AIDS epidemic. There are no aspects inherent to homosexuality that make male homosexuals uniquely susceptible to infection with HIV. Instead, the predominance of male homosexuals who suffer from AIDS in both the United States and Europe is attributable to the early arrival of HIV in the homosexual population and its dissemination by individuals with multiple sex partners. In the first few years of the AIDS epidemic, American homosexuals with AIDS were compared with American homosexuals without AIDS. The principal difference between the two groups was the much higher number of total lifetime and recent sex contacts in the group with AIDS than in the group without AIDS. Patients with AIDS averaged about 61 sex contacts in the preceding year, whereas those without AIDS averaged about 25 contacts over the same period.

The identification of HIV as the cause of AIDS explained the preponderance of male homosexuals early in the AIDS epidemic. Any group that has frequent sexual contacts amplifies the chance of spreading a sexually transmissible disease among its members. The frequency of contact with different sex partners increased the risk of HIV transmission among homosexual men, not the nature of the homosexual contact.

If another circumscribed population had some portion of its members infected with HIV but the group was unfailingly monogamous, HIV would not spread outside of the small number of individuals originally infected. This is also true for male homosexuals. If the individuals first infected entered monogamous relationships, then HIV infection would have been limited to those people first infected. The opposite occurred in both Europe and the United States. The individuals who first encountered HIV were infected because they had multiple sex partners and thereby amplified their risks of contacting an HIV-infected person. Once infected, they did not alter the practices that led them to become infected. They then unknowingly infected many other homosexuals with whom they had sex. It is not surprising that many of the first homosexuals with AIDS in the United States reported having over 1,000 different sex partners in their lifetime. This degree of sexual activity enhanced their chance of meeting an individual carrying HIV, even though the number of HIV-infected individuals was relatively low at that time. Therefore, the principal reason for the high incidence of AIDS in male homosexuals is the early arrival of HIV in that group, and its subsequent spread by those individuals who had many sex partners.

There is no reason to believe that male homosexuals are more at risk for infection than heterosexuals. Heterosexuals engaging in anal sex, oral sex, and other sex practices that provide exposure to infected body fluids are at the same risk of transmitting HIV from an infected partner to an uninfected partner as are homosexuals.

53. Can HIV be transmitted via oral sex?

There are many different forms of oral sex. Perhaps the most common form of oral sex is orogenital sex, contact between the mouth and the genitals.

Because individuals who engage in orogenital sex rarely do so to the exclusion of other forms of sexual contact, it is difficult to attribute transmission of HIV to oral sex and not to other types of sexual exposure. Nonetheless, some researchers have attempted to understand the risk of oral sex as a route of transmission of HIV by studying individuals who claim to have practiced solely oral sex for a several-month period before becoming infected with HIV. One study of a gay male population found several patients who became infected with HIV while claiming to practice only orogenital sex for at least six months before seroconversion. About one-half of the 20 seroconverters later admitted that they had also engaged in receptive anogenital intercourse in that same period, thereby raising some doubt to the consistent practice of only orogenital sex in the remainder of patients. Other case reports do exist that strongly implicate orogenital sex as a route of HIV transmission. The relative transmissibility of HIV by this route compared to other forms of sexual transmission is difficult to estimate.

Work with non-human primate models support orogenital sex as a mode of HIV transmission. Adult macaques exposed orally to solutions containing HIV were readily infected with the virus at about 1/6000 the viral inoculum necessary to infect the animals via the rectal route. How the virus engages target cells through the mouth is unclear, although periodontal disease, mucosal portals, the tonsils, and the surface of the stomach are logical possibilities.

The role of orogenital sex as a route of transmission of HIV is, at best, poorly studied in populations other than in homosexual men. The possibility of transmitting HIV from the vagina to the mouth seems possible, although it is not documented. Similarly, the feasibility of transmitting HIV from the mouth to the genitals is unclear. One can speculate about plausible routes of transmission in any type of orogenital contact. HIV-bearing lymphocytes present in semen could contact damaged mucous membranes in the mouth, and allow the entry of HIV into tissue. Likewise, traces of menstrual blood or vaginal discharges containing HIV could serve as conduits of infection from the genitals to the mouth. The shedding of virus in the mouth is also a theoretical source of HIV transmission to the genitals, whether male or female, but convincing documentation of this route of infection is lacking.

Despite limitations in assessing the risk, orogenital sex should be considered a possible means of transmitting HIV. This caution is underscored by a study that evaluated 46 adults with recent HIV infection. Four of the patients reported having only unprotected oral-genital contact during a single sexual encounter believed to be the cause of their HIV infection.

54. How is HIV transmitted via blood?

HIV reproduces in CD4 lymphocytes that circulate in the blood and other body fluids. Blood collected for transfusion contains these lymphocytes. Even if it were possible to remove every lymphocyte from blood before it was transfused into another person, it would be impossible to eliminate all of the HIV.

HIV is not only associated with the cells in which it grows, but it also is present in blood unassociated with cells. Thus, introduction of blood from an infected person into an uninfected person will transfer both small numbers of lymphocytes and free virus to the transfusion recipient.

Of all the forms of exposure to HIV, blood transfusion is the most efficient means of transferring virus from one person to another. No barriers of any kind exist between the infected person and the individual who receives contaminated blood directly into his or her bloodstream.

Contaminated blood plays a central role in the transmission of HIV well beyond just those cases resulting from the transfusion of tainted blood. Any contaminated blood introduced into a person's bloodstream is a potential route of transmission of HIV. Blood contaminating medical equipment such as scalpels or other sharp objects, blood lining a needle used by an addict to inject drugs, and glass vials containing blood that break and pierce the skin are all demonstrated routes by which HIV can infect a person.

On the other hand, exposure to the small cuts and abrasions that may develop during the practice of many sports has not led to HIV infection. These circumstances must be considered potential routes of transmission, but common sense should dictate the degree of risk that actually exists in a given set of circumstances.

55. What is the risk of being infected with HIV via a blood transfusion?

The risk of acquiring HIV from appropriately screened transfused blood is very low. The fraction of all cases attributable to infection by this route has decreased in developed countries. This decline is attributable to the uniform institution of practices designed to avoid the introduction of HIV into the blood supply. Two practices are fundamental in eliminating HIV from the blood supply: voluntary deferral of those at risk for HIV infection from blood donation and laboratory screening of all donated blood for evidence of HIV.

Refusing blood donations from those at risk for HIV infection, and the widespread use of screening for HIV, have dramatically reduced the chances of acquiring HIV from transfused blood. Since the introduction of screening tests in 1985, about 40 cases of transfusion-related HIV infection have occurred in the United States. It is estimated that among the 12 million blood donations currently collected every year in the United States, between 18 to 27 HIV-infected donations (one in 450,000 to 660,000 donations) are available for transfusion.

The uniform screening of all donated blood for the presence of HIV began after March 2, 1985. On that date, the United States Food and Drug Administration licensed the first screening test to detect antibodies against HIV in blood. Within one month, virtually all blood bank centers in the United States were using this technique. Initial results found that 0.25% (one in 400) of the first 1,100,000 units of donated blood collected in 131 blood centers in the United States between April and June 1985 were HIV infected. After a campaign to discourage high-risk individuals from donating blood, studies now find that less than 0.01% (one in ten thousand) individuals presenting themselves for donation are HIV infected. All of the units found to be infected are routinely discarded.

The United States Public Health Service recommends that blood banks confidentially notify donors of blood found to be infected. The Public Health Service also recommends that the donor be referred to a physician for counseling and further medical evaluation including a review for risk factors and an examination for the presence of medical conditions consistent with HIV infection. Some prospective blood donors falsely believe that the act of donating blood may lead to infection with HIV, but there is no risk of infection by donating blood. All equipment is sterile and used only once. The only potential risk associated with blood donation lies with the transfusion of blood from a donor infected with HIV into another person.

Even though the risk of infection from blood transfusion approaches zero, two factors prevent the risk from decreasing completely to zero. First, the antibody test used to find HIV is highly accurate but does have a very low error rate. Second, individuals recently infected with HIV may not develop antibodies for a few weeks after infection. If these people do not know that they are at risk and do not produce antibody detectable by the screening test, they may donate blood and inadvertently infect others.

Despite these possible circumstances, the risk of HIV infection from a blood transfusion is exceedingly low. Patients who know that they will receive blood, however, may further reduce the low risk of HIV infection by banking their own blood in advance of a scheduled surgical procedure. In this case, they will receive only their own blood if a transfusion is required. For the many patients who are unable to donate their own blood, the risk-benefit balance falls clearly on the side of receiving a transfusion when blood is medically warranted.

56. Who should not donate blood?

The CDC, the Food and Drug Administration, and blood banking organizations advise the following groups to refrain from the donation of blood and plasma:

- People with clinical or laboratory evidence of HIV infection
- Anyone who has ever used a needle for self-injection of drugs not prescribed by a physician
- Men who have had sexual contact of any kind with another male, even once, since 1977

- People who have accepted money or drugs in exchange for sex anytime since 1977
- People who have received clotting factor concentrates for diseases such as hemophilia
- Individuals who have had sexual contact of any kind, even once, with any member of the above groups

57. Do other blood products transmit HIV?

Blood products used in traditional ways, including for transfusion and the replacement of deficient blood-clotting proteins, are subjected to rigorous screening programs to remove tainted blood. The risk of acquiring HIV from these products is exceedingly low. Another product recovered from blood is used to produce the vaccine that prevents hepatitis B virus infections. The procedures used to prepare the compound inactivate any potentially contaminating virus. In addition, a second vaccine that does not use human material is available for use. Pooled antibody preparations, or immunoglobulins, also are derived from blood. This material also is exposed routinely to rigorous chemical procedures that thoroughly inactivate virus; no cases of HIV infection have been linked to use of immunoglobulins despite their widespread use.

Untraditional and untested products may not have the same low risk for HIV transmission found in those compounds that have been developed under conditions designed to inactivate HIV. For example, in 1985 the CDC reported that a private clinic in the Bahamas had offered cancer patients vials of human serum not approved for use in the United States. This unproved cancer therapy, termed immunoaugmentative therapy, consisted of injecting tumor proteins and blood from a large number of volunteers into patients. In May 1985, HIV was recovered in some of the material used for injection and the clinic closed two months later.

58. How do intravenous drugs figure in the transmission of HIV?

Intravenous drug users are a crucial link in the introduction of HIV into increasingly wider segments of the population. Intravenous drug use is a route of transmission of HIV because drug users frequently share the paraphernalia used to inject drugs. Small volumes of contaminated blood remain inside used paraphernalia such as needles and syringes, and can transmit HIV.

In the early years of the epidemic, studies found that many intravenous drug users were male homosexuals who were already infected with HIV. These individuals facilitated the introduction of HIV into the intravenous drug-using population and then to the sex partners of the drug users. In 1990 an estimated 1.1 million Americans injected illicit drugs and over 80% of them were believed to share needles. By 1992, the highest rate of increase in AIDS incidence in New York City was among female injecting drug users. In 1996, injecting drug use remained a major means of unabated HIV transmission, and in the United States is the risk behavior most frequently associated with heterosexual and perinatal transmission of HIV.

Much has been learned about the spread of HIV in the drug-using population. Because of the early widespread arrival of HIV in intravenous drug users in New York City, this population served as a model for transmission of HIV through drug use. Studies conducted in New York found that up to 88% of infected drug users admitted to routinely sharing needles with other drug users. Early in the AIDS epidemic, 74% of New York City intravenous drug users claimed to frequent shooting galleries, sites where needles are passed widely among anonymous drug users. Many that did not attend shooting galleries often used drug injecting equipment provided by their drug dealer, who also lent the same equipment to others. About one-half of New York City drug users who acquired HIV early in the AIDS epidemic knew that they had shared needles with homosexual men. Although this implies a significant introduction of HIV from male homosexuals into the population of drug users, the majority of drug users are heterosexual. Heterosexuals likely further spread the virus into groups who never have had contact with male homosexuals.

Although the transmission of HIV in drug users in the New York City metropolitan area is well studied, New York is by no means the only area where this form of transmission is important. Rapid increases in the prevalence of HIV in drug users in major urban areas from around the world were recorded in the late 1980s and early 1990s. Large geographic bands that follow the major transportation routes of heroin and cocaine roughly delineate where HIV infection in drug users is most severe. These areas include a swath across Southern Europe from Spain to the area that included the former Yugoslavia, a stretch in Asia from southern China to northern India, and a large part of Brazil.

59. Can HIV transmission by intravenous drug users be reduced?

Only completely avoiding exposure to contaminated blood will prevent infection with HIV while injecting drugs. In many cases, drug users do not take adequate precautions by using sterile injecting equipment. Public health measures that have been set up in different cities have reduced the risk of HIV infection to varying degrees. Efforts to reduce HIV transmission among drug users include: offering educational programs that explain the risks inherent in using contaminated equipment; exchanging clean needles for used needles and syringes; legalizing syringe sales; providing antiseptics to treat needles before their use; implementing methadone maintenance programs; and providing primary drug treatment to wean the individual from his or her habit. No single approach is uniformly effective and the relative values of each of those different procedures is under evaluation.

In particular, studies looking at the impact of needle and syringe exchange programs suggest that such programs decrease the use of needle and syringe sharing and other drug-risk behaviors. Available data do not support the hypothesis that such exchange programs increase drug use by increasing frequency of injection or by recruiting new users.

60. How is HIV passed to children and adolescents?

Over 90% of AIDS cases in children less than 13 years of age are a result of perinatal transmission from an infected mother to her child either during the pregnancy, delivery, or in the interval shortly after birth. Clinical studies demonstrate the presence of HIV in fetuses well before delivery, in umbilical cord blood obtained from the placenta, and in maternal blood lost during delivery. Exposure to any of these sources of virus is a potential route of transmission of virus.

The relative risks and rates of transmission through many of these routes remains an area of intensive study. The risk of perinatal transmission of HIV without therapeutic intervention is estimated to be about 25%, and this risk is greatest in women with advanced HIV disease, high levels of plasma HIV, and events that increase fetal exposure to maternal blood during labor and delivery. These observations and the beneficial effects of antiretroviral (zidovudine) therapy in reducing maternal-to-fetal HIV-1 transmission, suggest that the amount of HIV present in maternal blood (termed viral load) and events that increase exposure of the fetus to this blood, are the crucial determinants of the risk of HIV transmission. The use of zidovudine during pregnancy followed by brief treatment of the newborn infant reduces the risk of neonatal infection by about two-thirds, to an overall rate of less than 10%. The CDC now recommends that zidovudine be used in selected women who are pregnant and HIV infected, to reduce the risk of maternal-to-fetal transmission.

Children and adolescents are also susceptible to HIV infection through any of the routes commonly encountered in adults, including drug use and sexual activity. As of 1996, adolescents between 13 and 19 years of age comprise one of the most rapidly growing populations of AIDS cases. Of the 4,221 patients in this category, sexual contact was the major means of acquiring HIV infection.

Young children who are not sexually active are also at risk for sexual transmission of HIV. One research team found a high incidence of sexual abuse in a group of children with HIV infection. Of 96 HIV-infected children aged 3.5 to 13 years, 14 suffered sexual abuse and 4 were exposed to HIV by this route. HIV infection in a young child without an obvious maternal source should prompt at least consideration of the possibility of child abuse.

61. Is HIV transmitted by breast-feeding?

HIV has been isolated from the breast milk of infected women. A few case reports demonstrate that HIV is also transmissible through the milk of an infected woman to her breast-fed child. Physicians estimate the risk of transmission via breast milk at 29% for mothers who are postnatally infected. The risk is even higher for women who are infected prenatally—by as much as 14% beyond the risk of transmission *in utero* or during delivery.

The World Health Organization (WHO) and the United Nations Children's Fund recommend breast feeding for infants of HIV-infected women living in areas where infectious diseases and malnutrition are major causes of infant disease (i.e., in most developing countries). However, where malnutrition and infection are not major causes of infant mortality (e.g., in most developed nations), formula feeding is advised for HIV-infected women.

62. Why are hemophiliacs at risk for HIV infection?

As AIDS cases accumulated in the early 1980s, hemophiliacs were found to be a principal group at risk for the disease. They were at extremely high risk to encounter a blood-borne pathogen because of their frequent blood transfusions and use of clotting factor.

The early appearance of AIDS in both hemophiliacs and intravenous drug users implied that the illness was caused by some sort of agent transmissible through blood and helped to stimulate the search for a virus. The blood-borne link of a transmissible agent was further supported by an increasing risk of AIDS in people who had a greater number of exposures to blood products. Not all hemophiliacs had the same risk for HIV infection; hemophiliacs who had received few transfusions or had used cryoprecipitate, a product that provides clotting factors but is supplied by a small number of donors, had lower rates of HIV infection than those who received more blood products.

Hemophiliacs are born with an inherited bleeding disorder and are almost exclusively male. The disorder is determined genetically and results in poor blood clotting because of the absence of a single protein, or clotting factor, involved in coagulation. Various forms of hemophilia exist; hemophilia A (factor VIII deficiency) is usually the most severe, followed by hemophilia B (factor IX deficiency), and other types. In the past, hemophiliacs faced a markedly shortened life filled with a multitude of bleeding complications. That dismal prognosis improved with the introduction of concentrated clotting factor to replace the defective protein. By injecting the clotting factor, a hemophiliac can normalize blood coagulation. The factor is administered from vials containing clotting proteins from the blood of between 2500 and 25,000 donors.

As early as 1984 a CDC survey found about 74% of type A hemophiliacs were infected with HIV; about 39% of type B hemophiliacs were HIV infected. There has been no significant increase in these infection rates as a result of modifications made to the procedure to prepare clotting factors. Because heat treatment neutralizes the virus during factor preparation, the National Hemophilia Foundation recommends its use in place of the previous procedure.

The most prominent modification to the factors given to people with hemophilia is the systematic exclusion of HIV-infected donors by screening and donor self exclusion. The use of proven physical and chemical means that disrupt the virus and thereby render it noninfectious have reduced the risk of getting HIV from the products used to treat hemophilia to almost zero. Withholding therapy now poses a greater risk to patients than receiving properly processed clotting factors.

In 1989 the Medical and Scientific Advisory Council of the National Hemophilia Foundation released revised guidelines for the therapy of hemophilia to reduce the transmission of HIV. Recommendations were, in part, that:

- Factor VIII products be heated for 10 hours at 60°C; or are detergent-solvent treated; or monoclonal antibody purified; or heated in suspension in organic media; or dry heated at high temperatures.
- Viral-attenuated factor IX concentrate be treated with the methods described above for patients with factor IX deficiency.
- Fresh frozen plasma, a blood product containing clotting proteins, be used in factor IX deficiency with mild to moderate factor deficiency.
- Desmopressin (DDAVP), a synthetic hormone that improves clotting, should be used when possible with mild to moderate Hemophilia type A.
- Persons with von Willebrand's Disease (a different form of factor VIII clotting disorder) should be treated with DDAVP or cryoprecipitate from carefully tested donors. Patients with severe disease should receive processed factor VIII.

- Bleeding episodes should continue to be treated with the appropriate clotting factor.

AIDS now exceeds bleeding as the leading cause of death in people with hemophiliac. The continued development of improved procedures to inactivate HIV while not affecting clotting factor, the exclusion of persons at high risk for HIV infection from blood donation, and the diligent use of the HIV antibody test to identify blood from infected individuals, remain necessary steps if people with hemophilia are to avoid HIV during injections of clotting factors.

63. Do insects transmit HIV?

There is no evidence that HIV is spread from human to human by anything other than through blood, blood products, perinatal contact between mother and child, or sexual contact. One can attempt to imagine situations in which exposure to HIV by these means can occur without knowledge that an exposure is taking place, and insect bites may seem a reasonable scenario. If this were the case, one would expect AIDS in household members of persons with AIDS unrelated to sexual contact or at-risk behaviors. In addition, young children, other than those in risk groups, are frequently bitten by insects and should constitute a significant infected group if insect transmission takes place. There are no cases reported which clearly fit either of these situations.

An outbreak of AIDS cases in Belle Glade, Florida between 1982 and 1986 was first thought to implicate insects in the transmission of HIV. This agricultural community in western Palm Beach County was frequented by migrant farm workers who harvested sugar cane. It had many climatologic characteristics that seemingly favored an insect mode of transmission, if that route was viable. Health workers calculated that the incidence of HIV infection in Belle Glade was about 30 times higher than that expected for a comparable community in the United States with about 6% of the community between the ages of 18 and 29 infected with HIV. The high incidence of HIV in Belle Glade and its proximity to swamps suggested to some that mosquitoes transmitted HIV.

Federal researchers extensively investigated the outbreak of AIDS in Belle Glade. They found that all of the children infected were offspring of women who also were infected. No children were found to be infected other than those born to already infected women. Nearly all of the infected adults were members of groups known to be at high risk for HIV infection, while the few remaining adults without an identified risk behavior died before they could be interviewed. Finally, other laboratory tests assessing exposure to mosquitoes failed to implicate insect-borne HIV transmission. The researchers concluded that the high incidence of AIDS in Belle Glade was not due to biting insects, but was instead the result of recognized risk factors that were present at high levels in the population of that community.

Researchers have created laboratory circumstances to determine if insects can carry HIV. Scientists isolated HIV genetic material from bedbugs and mosquitoes one hour after feeding the insects blood contaminated with HIV, but the isolated virus did not grow in the insects' cells. The very low levels of HIV in blood, the tiny volumes ingested by insects and the absence of field data implicating spread of HIV by insects makes this form of transmission highly unlikely.

64. How can one reduce the sexual transmission of HIV?

The simplest way to avoid exposure to HIV is to limit sexual contacts with others. Because HIV is a retrovirus that leads to lifelong infection, sexual contact with new partners exposes one to the cumulative risks of HIV infection of all of the previous sex partners of the new individual.

The high prevalence of HIV infection in homosexual men illustrates this point. In this group, the rapid rate of exposure to new sex partners allowed individuals infected with HIV to spread the virus very quickly. If each infected person had ten new sex partners in a month, and if each of these new sex partners became infected and behaved similarly, then after only two months over one hundred new infections would occur. Each of the newly infected ten individuals would carry the virus and spread it to others as if the new partners were exposed directly to the person first infected.

The difficulty of identifying an infected person without testing is formidable. Several studies underscore this point by demonstrating that college-aged students were unable to identify the risk of their sex partners. Two separate studies found that the majority of men and women who were sexually active did not realize that their partners had been involved sexually with a total of more than one person previously. Many female partners of infected bisexual men had no idea that their partner was bisexual.

Only HIV antibody testing can reliably identify infected people if they do not voluntarily reveal their risk status. Even the antibody test is imperfect; new sex partners may have become infected only recently and not had sufficient time elapse to allow the production of antibodies detectable by the test.

Public health officials now recommend safer sex practices to reduce the risk of infection with HIV. These practices apply to sex with new partners and are also useful in guiding the sexual practices of people already known to be infected with HIV. Reports that up to 75% of adolescents engage in sexual intercourse by 19 years of age emphasizes the extent of the risk in even the youngest age groups. The most effective procedures in safer sex avoid direct contact with any potentially infectious body fluids by the use of barriers such as condoms.

65. What is safe sex?

It is impossible to create an exhaustive list of different sex acts and assign each a relative risk of infection from HIV. The desire to determine what constitutes "safer sex" led to a list that attempts to link risks to a variety of sex practices. This list, shown in Figure 4-5, as in all others, combines what is known to be true with what seems reasonable based on the state of knowledge today.

Figure 4-5: HIV transmission risks for different sex practices

Unsafe Practices with High Risk of HIV Transmission

- Numerous sex partners
- Unprotected anal receptive sex with an infected partner
- Unprotected anal penetration with the hand ("fisting")
- Anal douching in combination with anal sex
- Oral-anal contact
- Vaginal intercourse without a condom with an infected partner

Possibly Unsafe Practices with Unclear Risk of HIV Transmission

- Fellatio (oral contact with male genitals and with semen)
- Cunnilingus (oral contact with female genitals)
- Sharing sex toys and implements

Low Risk Practices with Some Risk of HIV Transmission

- Anal or vaginal sex with proper use of intact condom
- Wet kissing (French kissing)
- Fellatio interruptus (contact with male genitals without ejaculation)

Practices with Probably No Risk of HIV Transmission

- Abstention from sexual contact
- Monogamous relationship, both partners uninfected
- Self masturbation
- Masturbation of partner (if no broken skin on hands and genitals of either partner)
- Touching, massage, hugging, stroking
- Dry kissing ("social kissing")

66. What is the evidence that these safe-sex practices are effective?

Multiple studies of homosexual men in San Francisco and New York City have shown a dramatic reduction of the number of sex partners since the beginning of the AIDS epidemic. With a declining number of sex partners, the rate of new infections has decreased in this group. The reduction in the number of sex partners also is reflected by decreased rates of other sexually transmitted diseases in the male homosexual population in some cities. However, other studies find that although many gay men report behavior changes reducing the chances of infection, after several months a significant proportion return to their original high-risk behaviors.

Homosexual groups have achieved significant reduction in many risk behaviors. There is little evidence, however, that risk behaviors have been reduced substantially in heterosexuals or in intravenous drug users. Sexually transmitted disease clinics across the United States continue to observe an epidemic of sexually transmitted diseases among heterosexuals including syphilis and genital herpes. Many drug users continue to avoid using sterile needles before injecting drugs. In addition, the association of promiscuity and the use of intravenous drugs continues to place many at risk for HIV infection.

There are, however, some positive findings scattered across different populations. One study evaluated college women from three separate years who consulted gynecologists at a university health care center in either 1975, 1986, or 1989. The study found no differences in the number of sex partners or frequency of intercourse among women in these three groups over the years in the study. The proportion of these women whose sex partners used condoms, however, increased from 12% to 41% in 1975 and 1989, respectively. The trend to use condoms was attributed to fear of HIV infection and an increased general awareness among people in this age range that they are at risk for infection with HIV.

A simple example illustrates the importance of following safe sex practices. Assume that an uninfected homosexual has 40 sex contacts per year. If he lives in a city such as Seattle which has a gay population where one in every three homosexuals is infected with HIV, then after forty different random contacts, the person would almost certainly be exposed to HIV. If this person reduced the number of new sex contacts by 90% to a total of four new sex contacts, then the risk of infection would fall, but not significantly. This person would still have about an 80% chance of contacting someone who was HIV-infected if new sex partners were selected randomly. Although the probability of interacting with someone who is infected with HIV is determined by the population in which one moves, reducing the number of sex partners is an important first step to lower the probability of encountering a partner infected with HIV. Safe sex practices, however, provide the greatest reduction of risk by completely avoiding contact with infectious material.

A large study of heterosexuals in Thailand demonstrated the importance of reducing the number of sexual contacts and employing safe sex measures. Thailand is confronting an explosive growth in prevalence of HIV infection. In 1990, the Ministry of Public Health began an educational program to promote the use of condoms among customers of sex workers. Five specific groups of young men (4,311 men total) were evaluated between 1991 and 1995. In the 1991 and 1993 groups, the prevalence of HIV infection was around 10%. In the 1995 group, the prevalence decreased to around 6%. This reduction in seroprevalence was associated with a decreased proportion of the men reporting sexual contact with a sex worker, and an increased proportion of the men reporting use of condoms during sexual contact with sex workers. Avoidance of risk behaviors from HIV transmission and use of barrier methods remain the most effects means of reducing HIV infection.

67. Are condoms, diaphragms, and spermicides effective in preventing HIV transmission?

There is evidence that latex condoms offer significant, but not absolute, protection against HIV transmission. Latex condoms tested in the laboratory under conditions designed to simulate intercourse consistently prevent the passage of HIV. Natural materials such as lamb intestine used in some condoms do not perform well in these tests and are not recommended to prevent HIV infection. The laboratory setting cannot simulate all of the conditions encountered during the use of condoms and these studies cannot be considered conclusive evidence that condoms will unfailingly prevent HIV transmission. Condoms also may break due to improper storage, use, and other factors that cannot be assessed in laboratory settings.

The difficulty of extrapolating laboratory results to actual experience is demonstrated by data collected during studies of the success of condoms when used for contraception. As is the case with HIV, condoms are effective in preventing the passage of sperm, although partners using condoms as contraception have annualized pregnancy rates of 10%. Although condoms do not provide perfect protection, the most important determinants of success with condoms is their diligent and proper use. Studies indicate that the 12% of reproductive-age women in the general population who currently use condoms reduce the number of new HIV infections per year in the United States by up to 11% per year. The effectiveness of condoms in reducing HIV infection is further supported by a study of 304 HIV-negative individuals whose only risk factor for infection was a monogamous relationship with an HIV-infected partner. After an average of 20 months, and an estimated 15,000 total episodes of intercourse, 124 couples reported using condoms consistently. None of the uninfected partners from these 124 couples became infected with HIV, in contrast with many of those individuals who did not consistently use condoms.

Diaphragms and cervical caps also seem to hold some promise in preventing the transmission of HIV. These devices have not been rigorously tested, but epidemiological studies show a reduced incidence of other sexually transmitted diseases in women who use these devices. However, it is important to note that these devices cover only the cervix and do not raise a barrier over the surface of the vagina where HIV infection almost certainly takes place with greatest frequency. These devices cannot be considered protective against the spread of HIV.

Female condoms are a polyurethane sheath with a pouch to accommodate the penis. The sheath covers both the cervix and the vagina. Although the device is available in the United States, data indicating that it prevents the transmission of HIV are still accumulating. Because the annualized pregnancy rate of couples using only this form of contraception is about 15%, it seems that this device will reduce but not provide complete protection against HIV transmission. This is one of the very few products that allows a female partner to determine the use of a barrier contraception that might markedly reduce HIV infection.

Spermicides such as nonoxynol-9 have been recommended as a means to reduce the likelihood of HIV transmission, but no controlled study has demonstrated yet that this agent alone reduces the transmission of HIV. It seems unlikely that substituting a spermicide for a barrier form of contraception will prevent transmission of HIV if one partner refuses to use a condom.

68. How can one minimize the risk of HIV transmission with condoms?

HIV transmission, despite condom use, is rarely attributable to a failure of the condom itself and is more often attributable to their incorrect use. Three principal types of condom failure occur: breakage, leakage and improper use. Each of these types of failure can be minimized by the following techniques.

- Use a new condom for each act of intercourse.
- Use latex and not lambskin condoms.
- Use only fresh condoms. Condoms stored in cool, dark environments can last for many months to years. Significant deterioration occurs when condoms are exposed to light, temperatures over 100° Fahrenheit, or high humidity. Condoms should be removed from the wrapper only at the time of use.
- Use a lubricant or prelubricated condoms. Water-based lubricants such as K-Y jelly decrease the likelihood of breaking the condom. Oil-based products, including petroleum jelly and vegetable oil that are contained in many commercial products, can cause the deterioration and breakage of latex in as little as several minutes. One should confirm that the lubricant is safe when used with latex condoms by carefully reading the label of the lubricant to be used. Oil-based products should not be confused with water-based products because of a similar appearance or because they can washed off with water.
- The spermicide nonoxynol-9 should not be used alone for HIV protection. When used with a condom, it may increase the protection afforded by the condom. Some women may be sensitive to nonoxynol-9 and this may cause genital irritation and ulceration that could, without condom use, theoretically increase the risk of HIV infection.
- A proper condom should have a tip, bubble, or nipple at the end to collect semen.
- A condom should be worn as instructed on the product. It should not be unrolled until placed on the head of the penis.
- Condoms that feel gritty or gummy should not be used; the latex may have deteriorated.
- The condom should be held at the base of the penis immediately after ejaculation to prevent the condom from slipping while withdrawing the penis.

69. What is nonoxynol-9?

Nonoxynol-9 is an ingredient found in many spermicidal contraceptive agents. It acts as a contraceptive by disrupting spermatozoa via its detergent characteristics. The observation that this commonly used spermicide also inhibited the growth of HIV in laboratory settings led to frequent recommendations advocating its use as a means to reduce the likelihood of transmitting HIV during sexual intercourse.

There is clear evidence from laboratory studies that nonoxynol-9 inhibits the growth of HIV. It is effective at concentrations as low as 0.05% when exposed to the virus for at least 60 seconds. Levels that are 100 times this concentration kill lymphocytes, but the concentration of nonoxynol-9 that is typically encountered in most products containing the spermicide are from 0.1% to 1%. These products are likely to achieve the necessary concentrations in the vagina when the agent is used to destroy HIV.

Because nonoxynol-9 was developed for use as a contraceptive agent, it has not undergone rigorous testing in clinical studies to assure that it is also effective at preventing HIV infection during sexual intercourse. Several small clinical studies have found an increased incidence of genital ulceration in both male and female prostitutes who frequently used products containing the spermicide. Evidence of tissue irritation at the site of application has been found in other studies and has raised the question of whether the irritation increases the risk of HIV infection. It is impossible, however, to extrapolate from studies where large amounts of the material was used frequently to individuals who use the material on a daily or less frequent basis.

Finally, there are no studies that indisputably demonstrate nonoxynol-9 prevents HIV infection when used by individuals engaging in sexual intercourse. The agent is considered safe to use under circumstances similar to its intended use as a contraceptive, but its safety and effectiveness in preventing HIV transmission in anal intercourse have also not been rigorously tested. At the present time, use of nonoxynol-9 alone should not be considered protective against HIV. Concurrent use of nonoxynol-9 with a latex condom, however, may provide added protection against HIV transmission.

70. What other precautions reduce the risk of HIV infection?

Sexual transmission is the primary route of HIV spread. For people who do not engage in sex with others at risk for HIV infection and who maintain monogamous relationships, the principal risk of exposure is through contact with contaminated blood. Outside of health care workers and intravenous drug users who confront daily possible exposure to the virus through their work or behaviors, most people can further reduce an already low risk by paying attention to a few simple procedures.

All people should avoid sharing razors, toothbrushes, and any other personal product that may contact infected body fluids. Tattoos and other procedures that pierce the skin also may pose a risk for infection. Any person subjecting himself to such a procedure should determine that the equipment is sterile. When visiting a health care worker, patients should expect that their physicians and dentists use only sterile equipment and wear clothing appropriate for the procedure being performed to avoid transmission of HIV from either a patient to a doctor or vice versa. Generally speaking, observing simple rules of accepted hygiene will prevent infection.

71. Can HIV be transmitted through routes other than blood and sex?

The finding that AIDS was caused by a virus prompted much public debate about the transmissibility of the virus during the conduct of daily activities. Particular concern was focused on casual contact as a means of transmitting HIV to household members, non-medical caretakers, and others who came into contact with HIV-infected people.

Casual contact includes touching and holding another person or breathing the same air as an infected person. It also includes eating food prepared by an infected person, sharing eating utensils, being exposed to coughs, and living in the same household as a person with HIV infection. Finally, casual contact includes participating in any other activity that does not include exposure to blood, saliva, vaginal secretions, semen, blood, or the mucous membranes of another. Aside from the lack of evidence to indicate transmission of HIV through any of these means, there is also no evidence that HIV is transmitted through the use of swimming pools, spas, hot tubs, or toilets used previously by an infected person. These findings are confirmed by studies involving a few thousand patients over months of direct nonsexual patient exposure by family members. Extended observation failed to detect any evidence of transmission of HIV.

The isolation of HIV from saliva does not imply a risk of transmitting HIV by casual contact. Early studies showed that HIV is detected in saliva only with difficulty; one of 83 samples provided by 71 infected men yielded virus in the largest study of this type. Very low levels of virus were found in the one positive sample. Other work has found that saliva contains factors, probably proteins, that are potent inhibitors of viral growth. Despite the absence of cases known to have been transmitted first by casual contact and secondly by kissing, the practice of careful oral hygiene and avoiding exposure of saliva to mucous membranes around those with HIV infection seems prudent.

Other activities not involving sexual exposure or contact with blood fail to transmit HIV. Infected food workers who practice normal hygiene present no risk to others. They should avoid food preparation, however, if open skin lesions are present. Adequately cleaned cardiopulmonary resuscitation mannequins, exposure to tears, and related activities present no demonstrated risk for transmission of HIV. Routine medical care, including dental care, presents no risk if all equipment used is properly sterilized.

72. What are the risks of HIV transmission in athletics?

While there is a theoretical risk of transmitting HIV from an infected athlete to an uninfected athlete during competition, experts believe that this risk is very low. The World Health Organization (WHO) issued a consensus statement in 1989 and concluded that no evidence existed to expect a risk of HIV transmission when infected persons participating in sports have no open wounds or lesions. For athletes with a bleeding wound or skin lesion, recommendations to cover such wounds during competition have been made with the realization that transmission to another athlete would likely require a similar wound or lesion to serve as a portal of entry for HIV. As of March 1996, the CDC notes that no documented case of HIV transmission has been identified during any athletic event in the United States. The risk of such an occurrence has been estimated by the CDC to be less than one in 1 million.

Over the past five years, several professional and amateur athletes have revealed their HIV status, such as the late tennis player Arthur Ashe, basketball player Magic Johnson, Olympic diver Greg Louganis, baseball player Glenn Burke, late hockey player Bill Goldsworthy, and boxers Tommy Morrison, Lamar Parks, and Ruben Palacios. Several prominent figure skaters, including John Curry, Rob McCall, and Nicole Lesh also disclosed their HIV-infected status.

The media's attention to these sports figures have had profound effects. First, public awareness of risk of transmission of HIV among athletes and non-athletes has been raised. Secondly, such attention has emphasized that athletes engage in similar risk behaviors as does the general population and that HIV education should focus primarily on off-the-field activities. Athletes also may be at additional risk by engaging in special high-risk behaviors, such as the two documented cases of body-builders who acquired HIV by using contaminated needles to inject anabolic steroids.

73. Are household members who care for AIDS patients at increased risk for HIV infection?

There are no reported cases of HIV infection related to casual contact in household members directly involved in the care of family members with AIDS. In a case that did not involve casual contact, the CDC reported the apparent transmission of HIV from an ill child to his mother. The two year-old boy became infected with HIV after transfusion of contaminated blood. He required involved medical care at home, including the maintenance of a chronically indwelling venous catheter that allowed direct access to his bloodstream. Because his mother delivered much of his care while he was home, she had multiple contacts with his blood, saliva, and feces. The mother did not recall any puncture injuries to her skin while caring for the child, but she did not routinely wear gloves while working with the child or handling his body fluids. The mother was documented to have no infection with HIV before beginning home care for the child. Her husband tested HIV negative and there were no other risk factors identified in her life. The CDC concluded that the woman most likely acquired HIV from her son while providing intensive nursing care involving contact with his blood.

This case is not casual contact and cannot be considered typical of the exposure that household members experience when caring for persons with AIDS at home. It strongly emphasizes, however, how important it is for health care workers to follow the CDC guidelines for exposure to or handling of potentially infectious body fluids. Wearing gloves when handling the blood or body fluids of HIV-infected patients is especially important.

74. What are the risks of transmitting HIV from a patient to a health care worker?

No health care worker has been reported with HIV infection through casual contact while taking care of infected patients.

There are undisputed reports of health care workers becoming infected with HIV after direct exposure to blood containing the virus through accidental needle-sticks during routine patient procedures. Studies including over 1,700 health care workers show that the average risk of infection following a needle-stick contaminated with HIV-infected blood is less than 0.4%. Needle-sticks or other exposures to large quantities of contaminated blood may lead to infection more frequently than in 0.4% of cases, but precise figures tied to these variables are lacking. The risk of infection is increased when a subject experiences a deep injury with a contaminated needle, when blood is visible on the instrument, when the needle was previously placed in the vein or artery of the source patient, or in cases in which the source patient dies within 60 days of the exposure. There is no evidence of viral transmission by coughing or by other exposures inherent to typical patient care not directly involving blood.

Epidemiological data indicate that the percentage of all health care workers with AIDS is not significantly different from the percentage of people with AIDS in the general population. Of those health care workers with HIV infection, over 90% have recognized risk behaviors. Work-related exposures to HIV are a genuine risk to this group, however. As of June 1996, the CDC reported that 51 health care workers in the United States were infected with HIV through documented occupational exposures, most involving a needlestick injury.

Health care workers are constantly exposed to potential sources of HIV during their work and must, therefore, assume that any patient at any time may be infected. Needlestick injuries and cuts of the skin are common occupational hazards for people who provide direct patient care. A survey of medical resident physicians and medical students in 1989 and 1990 found an average of two puncture injuries with exposure to patient blood per year. Of the 1196 reported exposures, 52 were from different patients all known to be infected with HIV. Another survey, published in 1995, reported that 48% of all graduating medical students recalled being exposed at least once to potentially infectious body fluids during their clinical rotations, and over half of these exposures were skin punctures. Precautions preventing contact with blood and transmission of HIV must be followed at all times and without exception during patient care.

75. What risks do patients have from HIV-infected physicians or other health care workers?

Health care workers are more likely to be infected by patients than patients are to be infected by health care workers. There is only one documented case of a health care worker, a dentist, transmitting HIV to a patient. Scientists believe that the widely publicized case involved five different patients. An extensive investigation showed that the strain of virus infecting the dentist and the patients was identical and that there was no evidence of other routes of transmission. The infections most likely occurred during the course of the dentist's routine care of patients, although the precise means of transmission remain unclear.

Several studies have examined the patients of infected health care workers and found no instances of transmission from a health care worker to a patient. These studies included 1174 patients of an HIV-infected surgeon over a 13-year period and 900 patients of an HIV-infected dentist over a five-year period.

Mandatory testing of health care workers is not warranted because of the low risk of transmission and the expense of conducting a screening program.

76. What are appropriate precautions for health care workers to use with patients?

The CDC and the Occupational Safety and Health Administration (OSHA) introduced "universal precautions" to emphasize that precautions must be taken when exposed to any blood. Because any patient could be infected, all blood must be treated as infected by any person handling or exposed to blood. These precautions also apply to other bodily fluids that are a potential source of HIV including semen, vaginal secretions, and tissue. Universal precautions include these practices:

- Hand washing with soap and water between each patient contact.
- Use of disposable gloves if body fluids are contacted and double gloves during surgical procedures. Those with open skin lesions should not perform procedures if they are exposed to body fluids.
- Wearing of gowns when clothes may be exposed to body fluids.
- Wearing of masks and eyewear when performing procedures that may splash the worker with body fluids.
- Disposal of sharp instruments in puncture-resistant containers immediately after use. Needles should be disposed immediately after use without recapping. Disposal containers should be placed in all areas where sharp objects are used.

A pregnant health care worker limiting her interaction with HIV-infected persons to casual contact runs no increased risk of HIV infection for either herself or the fetus. Patients with AIDS are infected with other microorganisms such as cytomegalovirus that are more readily transmissible than HIV. The possible transmission of these other agents prompts recommendations that pregnant health care workers, without prior exposure and antibodies to these microorganisms, limit their exposure to AIDS patients and avoid direct involvement in their care.

77. What are adequate disinfection procedures for materials used by an HIV-infected patient?

HIV is readily destroyed by heat treatment and exposure to disinfectants. Recommended procedures to inactivate virus include the following:

Medical instruments: These should be treated with chemical disinfectants such as household bleach, also known as sodium hypochlorite. Bleach diluted from 1:5 to 1:100 in water will inactivate virus on contact. Other acceptable disinfection procedures include glutaraldehyde treatment and autoclaving, a procedure limited to sites with adequate facilities.

Medical instruments that contact the eye: These materials should be treated with 3% hydrogen peroxide for at least five minutes. Other acceptable disinfectants are a 1:10 dilution of household bleach, 70% alcohol, or 70% isopropanol. These instruments should be rinsed in tap water before reuse.

Contact lenses: Virus in soft lenses is inactivated by treatment with standard hydrogen peroxide contact lens solutions and by heat disinfection at 172° F for at least ten minutes. Hydrogen peroxide will also inactivate virus in rigid gas permeable and hard contact lenses.

Linen, clothes, glassware, and utensils: Laundry and dishwashing cycles commonly used in hospital settings are adequate to inactivate HIV on these materials.

Hard surfaces exposed to blood: Exposure to household bleach diluted 1:10 in water will inactivate the virus and 70% alcohol will reduce the amount of HIV, but not destroy it during short exposures, on these surfaces.

78. Will mandatory testing of hospital patients protect hospital staff from infection with HIV?

A well-publicized debate has taken place over the merits of forcing all patients admitted to hospitals to undergo mandatory testing for HIV infection. This policy has been advocated by some to protect health care personnel from infection with agents transmitted through the blood of patients. This approach presumes that health care workers will take precautions around infected patients that they would not have taken if the patient were not known to be infected. It would also identify patients infected only with the pathogens that are actually sought. Other pathogens, most notably hepatitis B, would escape detection and continue to present a threat to health care workers. In addition, patients who tested falsely negative would not prompt appropriate precautions that would lower the risk of transmission of virus from the patient to the exposed health care workers.

A simple, cost-effective strategy that protects health care workers not only from HIV infection but also from other infectious agents does not use testing, but instead assumes that all patients may be infected. By raising the infection control standards to uniformly high levels that prevent exposure to blood regardless of the results of screening tests, physicians can greatly reduce the risk of exposure to any blood-borne pathogen to levels lower than would be the case if precautions were taken solely on the basis of a laboratory result.

—CHAPTER FIVE—

The Diagnosis of HIV Infection

79. How is HIV infection diagnosed?

The diagnosis of HIV infection is made in four different fashions. The most time-consuming and least available method is the isolation and growth of virus in the laboratory from blood or other infected fluids and tissues. This procedure usually is not performed in hospitals unless the laboratory in that hospital isolates HIV for other research purposes.

A second way to detect virus is through the use of assays that directly measure the quantity of HIV RNA present in the bloodstream. These assays, called polymerase chain reaction (PCR) and branched DNA (bDNA), are highly sensitive and reproducible tools. Their use relies on the presence of RNA, a form of nucleic acid present in each virus particle. These highly sensitive assays are not typically used for diagnostic purposes, mainly due to their recent introduction as well as their cost.

A third way to detect the presence of HIV is through the body's response to the virus. The most common response is the production of antibodies directed against HIV. Tests that detect these antibodies are inexpensive and readily available to all qualified medical laboratories.

The final method to diagnose HIV infection is to infer infection from the presence of characteristic symptoms. This technique was used before the wide availability of antibody diagnostic kits. It remains a frequent method of diagnosis in parts of the world where access to antibody tests and other techniques is limited. Strict clinical criteria are used to diagnose HIV infection when no laboratory tools are obtainable, but infection cannot be diagnosed when no symptoms are present. In many developing countries of the world, thousands and perhaps millions of asymptomatic individuals go undiagnosed.

80. When is virus isolated from patients?

The isolation of virus from the blood or any of its components is not a routine laboratory test; the technique is expensive and time consuming. In many cases, especially before the later stages of AIDS, virus is cultured from plasma, the cell-free portion of the blood, only with great difficulty although the isolation is improved by culturing the cellular fraction of blood. Today, viral isolation by growth of the virus in special conditions is being increasingly replaced by the use of PCR and bDNA testing which detect the presence and quantity of virus in blood with greater ease than by standard viral culture procedures.

Viral isolation is not considered the best technique for diagnostic purposes. Antibody detection is both less expensive and, in cases where virus is not easily cultured, more sensitive than other techniques including culture, PCR and bDNA. PCR and bDNA will gain increased acceptance as the tests become more readily available and affordable, but they are unlikely to replace antibody-based techniques for large-scale screening such as blood banking and other epidemiological purposes.

Measurement of virus levels by PCR, bDNA or culture does have utility in circumstances other than in diagnosing HIV infection. Researchers have established that the amount of HIV present in blood, otherwise known as the viral titer, correlates with the stage of disease. This work has used PCR and bDNA technologies. Viral titers provide information that is essential to assess a patient's response to therapy and likely clinical course.

In addition, analysis of HIV repeatedly isolated from the same individual during the course of infection and grown in culture identifies subtle changes that arise in the molecular structure that distinguish offspring viruses from the originally infecting virus. By comparing the molecular structure of viruses, scientists can determine characteristics that suggest resistance to certain therapies.

Culturing of HIV also is essential to teasing out the molecular events that take place in the body that lead to the production of antibodies and other elements of the immune response. Further studies in this regard may help to design a vaccine and provide information essential to the creation of new drugs.

81. What is the antibody test that is used to diagnose HIV infection?

Tests that detect the presence of antibodies directed against HIV are used frequently in developed countries. This test uses disrupted HIV that is immobilized on a surface and is called an ELISA or enzyme-linked immunosorbent assay. It tests blood and other body fluids with indicator solutions that detect the presence of antibodies directed against HIV. The entire test requires tiny volumes of solutions and is automated to yield highly accurate results with a minimal opportunity for human or other types of error.

Inaccurate results in this diagnostic test are possible. Antibodies elicited by other substances in the blood may be similar to the antibodies directed against HIV and cross-react in the ELISA test, falsely indicating the presence of HIV. Although other forms of experimental error may be introduced by the improper use of the test reagents, the careful performance of the test and appropriate use of confirmatory procedures make the ELISA test accurate in over 99.5% of cases.

There are two possible outcomes from an ELISA test: the ELISA will indicate either that antibodies against HIV are present or absent. In the case where no antibodies are found, either the person is not infected (true in the vast majority of these instances) or he or she has not yet generated antibodies detectable by the test after infection. If the ELISA indicates that antibodies against HIV are present, then either the antibodies are truly caused by infection with HIV or the test has found antibodies that are cross-reactive with HIV antibodies, but there is no HIV present. Only further testing by using a Western blot technique will distinguish between these possibilities. Individuals who produce antibodies against HIV are termed seropositive; those who do not produce those antibodies are seronegative.

82. What is the role of the Western blot test?

If an ELISA yields positive results, the Western blot is run as a confirmatory test. The ELISA is more sensitive than the Western blot in detecting antibodies reactive with HIV proteins or proteins that are similar to HIV proteins. It is the extreme sensitivity of ELISA that may falsely indicate that HIV is present. The Western blot is a less sensitive test than the ELISA and when used to confirm a positive ELISA, accurately indicates infection with HIV.

The Western blot relies on a slightly different approach than does the ELISA. Disrupted HIV proteins are separated by size along a surface. Human serum containing antibodies reactive with the HIV proteins will appear only in those regions of the surface where the HIV proteins also appear. This technique, in contrast with the ELISA, not only establishes that antibodies that react with HIV are present, but it also identifies the proteins with which the antibody reacts. The demonstration that antibodies are truly directed against HIV makes the Western blot confirmatory of HIV infection.

These two tests, the ELISA and the Western blot, are used in tandem to establish the presence or absence of HIV infection. The ELISA is highly accurate in finding that no antibodies against HIV are present; a negative ELISA rarely needs further testing. Of course, if insufficient time has elapsed after infection to allow the production of antibodies or if subsequent exposure to HIV takes place, the ELISA will need to be repeated. In those cases where an ELISA test is positive, further testing with the

Western blot is indicated. A negative Western blot rules out infection with HIV and a positive blot confirms infection with HIV. When the tests are used in this fashion, they are accurate well over 99% of the time.

83. What is an indeterminate Western blot?

There are some circumstances in which a Western blot is neither positive nor negative. These tests are called indeterminate because the antibody pattern is not interpretable. One circumstance that may cause an indeterminate result is testing early after infection but before an adequate spectrum of antibodies are produced. Indeterminate Western blots, regardless of the pattern of ELISA reactivity, are best interpreted by determining if the person is a member of an HIV-risk group. Persons who are not members of an HIV-risk group and who have no other identifiable reason to be infected with HIV can have indeterminate Western blots. Those who are in risk-group categories may have their indeterminate Western blot result reflect an early but incomplete antibody response to infection. This latter group of individuals will require repeat testing to clarify their status.

Blood donors with negative ELISAs but indeterminate Western blots were studied along with their respective blood recipients to determine the outcome of indeterminate tests. All individuals who received blood from these donors failed to show any evidence of infection with HIV either by ELISA testing or by other laboratory techniques through serial observations. Thus, Western blot tests that are indeterminate are found in the population of individuals who are at no risk of HIV infection. Individuals who fall into this group are highly unlikely to be infected with HIV.

84. Will an indeterminate Western blot in a member of a low risk group remain so indefinitely?

A set of 99 individuals with indeterminate Western blots but without risk factors for HIV infection had their blots repeated over many months to monitor any changes. After a median period of 14 months of observation, 92% had blot patterns that remained indeterminate and only 8% had become unambiguously negative. None of the 99 individuals showed any evidence of infection with either HIV-1 or HIV-2. Other studies have found a higher percentage of individuals who have Western blots that become negative in a similar observation period, but in most cases the majority of those with indeterminate results will not change the status of their Western blot test during the course of at least a year. People at risk for HIV infection are less likely to have continuously indeterminate Western blots and therefore warrant follow-up testing.

85. Are there any other kinds of HIV antibody tests available?

In 1996, the FDA approved an oral HIV-1 antibody test that uses a sample called an *oral mucosal transudate* that is obtained from the inside of the cheek rather than saliva. Although not widely used at present, FDA approval was based on evidence showing a greater than 99% accuracy when compared with results from blood samples.

Two HIV antibody home collection systems that use blood are also available in the United States. These systems use the same technology as standard HIV antibody tests. The ability of individuals to place a small drop of their own blood on a coded lab mailing card has been considered a means to encourage participation by the greatest number of people at risk. Participants in this testing call the test result center at a specified time to receive test results and educational counseling.

86. What is the interval between infection and seroconversion?

Case reports have found the period between initial HIV infection and the production of detectable antibodies is most often between one and six months. The current antibody-screening tests have become increasingly sensitive and recent studies of blood donors suggest that these tests detect seroconversion in an average of 25 days after infection. In over 90% of individuals, seroconversion occurs within 120 days after infection when the latest generation of screening tests are used. The use of more sensitive techniques, including p24 testing and PCR to detect the virus before the body produces antibodies, may shorten the period of detection of HIV infection substantially. These tests, however, are not routinely used during screening for HIV infection.

Uncommon instances exist in which more than six months elapse before antibody is produced. Controversy surrounds the frequency with which this occurs and the most appropriate procedures to find virus when infection is strongly suspected but the antibody test remains negative. Conversely, well-documented cases in which a known exposure to HIV took place but serial antibody testing and other laboratory methods to detect HIV have remained negative for years show that not all exposures to HIV lead to infection.

87. Who should be tested for HIV antibody?

Since 1992, the CDC has recommended voluntary testing for people who have engaged in high-risk behaviors, which includes those who have multiple partners, those who have unprotected sex (anal, vaginal or oral sexual activity), injection drug users who share needles, and partners of infected people. Because of changes in treatment for newborn infants born to HIV positive women, HIV antibody testing is now encouraged for pregnant women, and if they test positive, for their child upon birth.

Current protocols in the United States mandate that all organ, tissue, sperm, and blood be tested before donation. However, anyone who has engaged in high-risk behaviors for HIV infection should not donate organs, tissues, sperm, or blood.

Currently, there are many publicly funded testing sites that offer anonymous antibody testing, with pre- and post-test counseling, and education. At this time, most test sites screen for the HIV antibody, since tests to screen for the actual virus are not commercially available. The period between infection and detection of antibody has shortened because current antibody tests are more specific, so that a person exposed to HIV may sero-convert within a month after their exposure. It is likely that 90% of persons exposed to HIV will develop antibodies after three months. Thus, some individuals who consider themselves at high risk will test every three to six months, especially if they are engaging in high-risk behaviors. Because of the interval between infection and development of the antibody, any negative test for HIV antibodies in these people is therefore rendered uncertain if an exposure took place shortly before the test.

88. Who is required to be tested for HIV?

HIV antibody testing is federally mandated for all military, United States Job Corps, and Peace Corps applicants. In addition, certain foreign countries require HIV antibody testing as a condition of obtaining a travel visa. HIV antibody testing also remains a requirement for those who donate organs, tissues, sperm, or blood.

89. What is the prevalence of HIV antibody positivity among various groups?

One approach to gauge seropositivity rates has been to examine such rates by risk exposure as well as type of testing site. In

1996, the CDC released data based on approximately 2.4 million HIV antibody tests that were obtained during 1994 and reported to local state and health departments (Figure 5-1). Approximately 2% of all those who were tested had positive test results. Of those who were tested, 13.8% of homosexual or bisexual intravenous drug users had positive test results, and 1.3% of heterosexuals at risk had positive test results.

Although self-reporting of risk behaviors is anonymous, there is not independent verification that self-disclosure of behaviors at risk for HIV infection is accurate in this setting. The rates may also be affected by a variety of other reasons. Individuals presenting themselves for screening may have a strong reason to suspect that they may be infected. Others from the same risk group who do not hold the same belief and may be less likely to be infected may not present themselves for testing. If there is a difference in the individuals comprising these groups, the seropositivity rates may be either elevated or reduced by biases in the screened population. Nevertheless, these figures do help characterize in general terms the degree to which people are infected by risk exposure and identification by site type.

Figure 5-1: HIV tests by risk exposure and testing site type in the United States, 1994.

Risk Group	No. of Tests	Positive Tests No.	(%)	% of total tests	% of total positive
Homosexual/ bisexual IDU*	11,995	1,652	(13.8)	0.5	3.9
Homosexual/ bisexual	160,676	12,486	(7.8)	6.7	29.3
Heterosexual IDU	136,609	7,452	(5.5)	5.7	17.5
Hemophiliacs	134	3	(2.2)	0.0	0.0
Blood recipient	20,487	250	(1.2)	0.9	0.6
Heterosexuals at risk	906,395	12,067	(1.3)	37.8	28.4
Other	896,639	6,689	(0.7)	37.4	15.7
Unknown	262,860	1,963	(0.7)	11.0	4.6
Total	**2,395,795**	**42,562**	**(1.8)**	**100.0**	**100.0**

Type of Clinic	No. of Tests	Positive Tests No.	(%)	% of total tests	% of total positive
HIV Counseling/ Testing	739,395	15,067	(2.0)	30.8	35.4
STD**	672,784	11,204	(1.7)	28.0	26.3
Drug Treatment	115,847	3,741	(3.2)	4.8	8.8
Family Planning	285,686	875	(0.3)	11.9	2.1
Prenatal/Pregnancy	142,394	632	(0.4)	5.9	1.5
TB	16,625	428	(2.6)	0.7	1.0
Other health dept.	204,210	4,290	(2.1)	8.5	10.1
Prison	77,144	2,211	(2.9)	3.2	5.2
College	2,948	4	(0.1)	0.1	0.0
Private physician	20,863	617	(3.0)	0.9	1.4
Other	116,157	3,407	(2.9)	4.8	8.0
Unknown	5,476	146	(2.7)	0.2	0.3
Total	**2,399,529**	**42,622**	**(1.8)**	**100.0**	**100.0**

Several areas do not report all variables on each test (i.e., risk factors, sex, age, and race or ethnicity). Therefore, the totals in sections of the tables may differ.
* IDU = injecting drug user
** STD = sexually transmitted disease clinic

Statistics obtained from: *HIV counseling and testing in publicly funded sites: 1993-1994 summary report.* US Department of Health and Human Services. Atlanta: Centers for Disease Control and Prevention, March 1996.

90. Are asymptomatic seropositive individuals infectious to other people?

A person infected with HIV is infectious to others regardless of the presence or absence of symptoms. Antibody testing in the mid 1980s established the infectivity of carriers of HIV. Healthy blood donors retrospectively determined to be infected with HIV transmitted HIV to recipients of their blood before they were known to be infected. There is also evidence that semen contains HIV in asymptomatic individuals early in the course of their HIV infection.

Those who carry HIV unknowingly and without symptoms are the principal reservoir for HIV in all studied populations. The absence of symptoms in these people gives no clue to their sex partners, whether new or long-standing, of their risk for HIV infection. The transmission of the virus by infected asymptomatic carriers is responsible for sustaining and expanding the epidemic. In the median ten years before an AIDS-defining condition develops after HIV infection, an asymptomatic person need only infect one other person to sustain the epidemic, or more than one to expand the epidemic. Controlling transmission during the many years before people know that they are infected is probably the single most important factor to slowing and reversing the spread of the epidemic.

91. How can HIV infection be diagnosed in an infant?

The usual serologic procedures used to identify infection with HIV in adults are unreliable in recently born infants. Maternal antibodies, including those directed against HIV, are transported across the placenta before birth. The mother's antibodies may then be detectable in the child's blood and incorrectly indicate the child to be infected with HIV. Conversely, the absence of antibodies in an infant does not rule out infection with HIV. Procedures other than serology must be used to find HIV infection in infants before 18 months of age. At 18 months, maternal antibodies are no longer present and the child can generate his own antibodies.

The clinical course of a child may allow diagnosis of HIV infection before maternal antibodies disappear. In the absence of clinical AIDS, demonstration of the presence of HIV by viral culture, p24 antigen positivity or PCR technology can make the diagnosis. PCR is a highly sensitive laboratory technique used to detect HIV DNA or RNA. Many reports have found PCR to be a more sensitive assay than viral culture; both of these procedures are more sensitive than p24 antigen reactivity. As is the case with most diagnostic tests used for research purposes, viral culture and PCR may not be available at all hospitals.

92. Where can one receive HIV-antibody testing?

HIV-antibody testing is readily available at a variety of medical facilities. People considering HIV-antibody testing must consider the medical setting most satisfactory to their purposes. A known and trusted physician may be best suited for some persons; other individuals prefer the anonymity of a testing facility devoted to maintaining individual secrecy. Local health departments and AIDS hotlines (Appendices A and B) can provide the location of anonymous testing facilities. The nature and quality of counseling offered to those with positive test results will undoubtedly vary from facility to facility and from physician to physician. Recently, two FDA-approved HIV antibody home collection systems allow another means to determine one's HIV antibody status.

93. Is there a role for a mass screening program?

Some have advocated applying mandatory screening for HIV infection to large portions of the population. Advocates state that such an approach will identify large numbers of people who are currently infected but unaware of their infection. Knowledge of the presence of HIV could influence them to modify their behavior to reduce the risk of transmitting the virus to others who may be uninfected.

This has prompted much debate. Some who are opposed to the widespread screening, whether in the population at large or even within highly defined subgroups, believe that mandatory testing of people will drive those most in need of the testing results underground. Many fear that the results of their test might not be held confidential and that they may become social pariahs and risk losing friends, employment, and social station, and even perhaps face quarantine. The debate over how to respect civil liberties within the context of a public health crisis is not resolved. Other factors outside legal and social concerns must be included in the design of any policy for testing for HIV in the general population.

A positive antibody test result in a high prevalence group (intravenous drug users) is more likely to be accurate than a positive test result in a low prevalence group (nursing home residents). For example, assume two different populations in which the incidence of HIV infection is 1 per 500 in the first and 1 per 50,000 in the second. Also assume that the test falsely detects 1 in 5000 uninfected persons as antibody positive (> 99% accurate). In the first population the antibody test will be correct over 90% of the time that a positive test result is returned (100 true positives per 50,000 tested with 10 additional false positives). In the second population, the antibody test will be correct only about 10% of the time that a positive result is returned (1 true positive per 50,000 tested with 10 additional false positives). Therefore, the frequency with which a test accurately indicates infection is determined by the prevalence of infection in the tested group.

Any mass screening program is expensive and entails challenging logistics; the cost must be worth the benefit. For example, Illinois and Louisiana briefly had laws requiring HIV antibody testing for couples planning to marry. The laws were repealed after the diagnostic yield of the test was found to be very low. Only eight individuals in Illinois were found to be seropositive out of 70,846 screened in a six-month interval for a cost of about $312,000 per seropositive person. During the same time, the number of marriage licenses issued in the state decreased by 22.5% as many couples avoided the law by marrying in other states; as a result, state revenues dropped as well.

The United States military has used routine and mandatory HIV-antibody testing of new recruits since 1985 and denies entrance to the military for those found to be infected. Between October 1985 and December 1995, 4,743,399 military applicants were tested and 4,403 or approximately 1 per 1,000 recruits were found to be infected. The rate for military applicants is believed to be lower than the general population because infected recruits are denied entrance to the armed forces, and this process may exclude certain high-risk individuals from applying.

There are populations that may be especially suitable for generalized voluntary screening. Patients hospitalized for acute care in hospitals in the United States constitute a group with a high incidence of HIV infection. From September 1989 through October 1991, 9,286 of 195,829 specimens (4.7%) were positive for HIV-1 among patients admitted to 20 United States hospitals. This rate of infection, if applied to the entire hospitalized population between the ages of 15 and 54, would identify an estimated 100,000 otherwise unrecognized cases of infection. Estimates since 1991 suggest that patients hospitalized in acute care settings, especially in large urban areas, remain a group with significant rate of HIV infection. More recent studies have suggested that offering zidovudine treatment to pregnant women with HIV infection not only will decrease the number of cases of pediatric HIV infections, but can have a positive and profound impact on health care costs.

94. What issues may influence a mandatory testing program?

In 1986 the Institute of Medicine and the National Academy of Sciences examined this issue and concluded that mandatory HIV testing would not be useful. They found that some persons in high prevalence groups who engage in illegal behavior, such as the use of intravenous drugs, would not comply with a mandatory program. These individuals could go to great lengths to influence the result of their test and thereby invalidate its utility to themselves and to the agency doing the testing.

Programs based on sexual orientation also would not likely be useful. For example, a homosexual man who is monogamous is less likely to transmit HIV than is a heterosexual man with multiple sex partners. Identifying groups of persons based on sexual orientation for mandatory testing would be needlessly discriminatory and potentially inaccurate.

The mandatory testing of people from selected groups would need to be completed on a routine basis. While a positive result is unlikely to change, a negative result can change if a later infection takes place. Individuals who are seronegative on a test today and who continue risk behaviors may well become seropositive at some point in the future; therefore any group deemed appropriate for mass screening would require follow-up of some periodicity if seronegative on an initial test.

The final point made in the study was that identification of HIV infection did not guarantee that the individual would undertake the required changes in behavior to reduce the risk of transmitting the virus to another person. Mandatory testing in certain risk groups such as pregnant women have been recently raised by the realization that zidovudine can reduce the risk of maternal-fetal transmission of HIV, and this has become a source of significant public policy debate.

—CHAPTER SIX—

The Epidemiology of AIDS

95. Where does AIDS occur in the world?

HIV infection and AIDS are now found on every inhabited continent. Epidemics are periods or outbreaks of unusually high incidence of disease in a community or area. Because the virus continues to spread across the world, the epidemic stretches across the globe making it of pandemic proportions.

The World Health Organization (WHO) maintains the most complete statistics on HIV infection outside of the United States. As of July 1996, WHO had received official reports of 1,393,649 cases of AIDS from over 200 countries. Almost 36% of the reported cases originated in Africa, with another 36.7% of reported cases coming from the United States. At the same time, WHO also provided provisional data, estimating worldwide HIV seroprevalence to be around 17 million. Because of substantial under-reporting, the number of AIDS cases and persons with HIV infection greatly exceed these estimates and are thought to be around 6 and 20 million, respectively.

In 1996, the greatest number of European AIDS cases continued to be in France, Italy, Spain, Germany, and the United Kingdom. In the Americas, Canada, Brazil, and Mexico continue to have the largest number of cases outside of the United States. Case reports of AIDS in Australia, Thailand, Singapore, India, and Indonesia continue to increase substantially, with rapid rises in the number of new infections reported in Southeast Asia and India. African countries such as Ivory Coast, Ethiopia, Ghana, Kenya, Malawi, Uganda, Tanzania, Zaire, Zambia, and Zimbabwe continue to have significant numbers of reported AIDS cases.

96. What is the incidence of AIDS in representative countries throughout the world?

The accuracy of reporting AIDS cases varies greatly from country to country for many different reasons. Despite the incompleteness of reporting, the WHO maintains a tally of all cases reported to it. One way to put AIDS in perspective is to compare the increase in cases over the last few years in representative countries (Figure 6-1). As of July 1996, WHO released reports current through June of 1996. Some countries reported their cases

Figure 6-1: A comparison of the number of AIDS cases by country from 1992 to 1996.

Country	Cumulative AIDS Cases		
	Cases 1992	Cases 1996	Date of latest report
Americas			
Argentina	1,820	8,197	(3/96)
Brazil	31,364	79,908	(2/96)
Canada	6,889	13,291	(3/96)
Mexico	1,034	28,544	(3/96)
United States	253,448	513,486	(12/95)
Europe			
Denmark	1,072	1,866	(3/96)
France	21,407	41,058	(3/96)
Germany	8,893	14,518	(3/96)
Italy	4,783	33,304	(3/96)
Spain	14,991	38,393	(3/96)
United Kingdom	6,510	12,565	(3/96)
Africa and Southeast Asia			
India	242	2,095	(12/95)
Malawi	22,300	43,067	(3/96)
Tanzania	34,605	82,174	(12/95)
Thailand	2,141	22,135	(12/95)
Uganda	34,511	48,312	(3/96)
Zaire	18,186	29,434	(4/96)
Zimbabwe	12,514	41,298	(10/95)
Western Pacific and Australia			
Australia	4,170	5,883	(11/95)
Japan	538	1,062	(12/95)

at some point in 1995; others reported as recently as June of 1996. In every case, the rate of rise in reported AIDS cases from 1992 to 1996 was rapid and substantial.

In 1996, the WHO estimated the number of adults in different countries living with HIV at the end of 1994, the most recent time that epidemiological information was available (Figure 6-2).

Figure 6-2: WHO country-specific working estimates of adult HIV seroprevalence as of December 1994.

Country	Estimated adults living with HIV
Americas	
Bahamas	6,000
Brazil	550,000
Honduras	40,000
Mexico	200,000
United States	700,000
Europe	
Denmark	4,000
France	90,000
Germany	43,000
Italy	90,000
Netherlands	3,000
Spain	120,000
Sweden	3,000
Switzerland	12,000
United Kingdom	25,000
Africa and Southeast Asia	
Congo	80,000
India	1,750,000
Malawi	650,000
Nigeria	1,050,000
Tanzania	840,000
Thailand	700,000
Togo	150,000
Uganda	1,300,000
Zimbabwe	900,000
Western Pacific	
Australia	11,000
Cambodia	90,000
Japan	6,200
Malaysia	30,000
New Zealand	1,200

Because HIV infection (unlike AIDS) is not reportable to local and national health agencies, WHO uses several methods and data sources to estimate the current and future magnitude of the HIV pandemic. WHO incorporates official country figures made by national experts or AIDS programs when available. When these figures are not available, estimates of HIV infection are based upon several factors: HIV seroprevalence studies, reported AIDS cases, estimates of under-reporting, country's population, and primary modes of transmission.

These estimates of HIV infection are considered under-estimates, but are intended to give a picture of the global pandemic. These figures should be looked upon as strictly provisional because of the challenges of accurately evaluating HIV infection levels in various countries worldwide.

97. How does AIDS in underdeveloped countries contrast with AIDS in developed countries?

HIV transmission rates in the United States have slowed in recent years, and appear to be leveling, primarily due to a decrease in transmission between men.

Different patterns of infection are found throughout the world. Although the majority of cases in the United States and Europe have occurred in homosexual and bisexual men, this pattern is not typical for most developing countries. Africa, Thailand, and some areas in the Americas including the Dominican Republic and Puerto Rico have HIV spread predominantly through heterosexual routes, while in Italy and Spain intravenous drug use is the primary form of transmission of the virus. The pattern of infection in Latin America resembles the pattern in the United States with a large prevalence of HIV infection in homosexual and bisexual men, but with the percentage of cases in heterosexuals increasing. Scientists describe these patterns as two HIV-1 epidemics, with Figure 6-3 listing their components.

Figure 6-3: Two HIV-1 epidemics

	Epidemic 1	Epidemic 2
Location	West (U.S., Europe)	South (Africa, S.E. Asia, Latin America)
Number infected	1.5 million adults & children	15-20 million adults & children
Epidemic status	Plateau or decreasing	Increasing
Exposure route	Blood, rectal bleeding	Vaginal intercourse

98. What are the transmission trends for HIV internationally?

In Europe, HIV transmission through injection drug use has and continues to be a major route of transmission, with the highest incidence in Spain and Italy. Injection drug use is also responsible for the alarming increase in HIV infection occurring in Eastern Europe in countries such as Poland and Ukraine. Generally speaking, the proportion of gay/bisexual men with AIDS has continually decreased over the last ten years in Europe, which is due to a rapid increase of HIV infection among injecting drug users and a low but stable increase in the proportion of heterosexual cases. Gay men and injection drug users still account for the heaviest burden of the AIDS epidemic throughout Europe.

Outside the developed countries, some programs designed to limit the spread of HIV infection are in place. In some cases policies intended to limit the use of imported blood are in effect. Other countries attempt to reduce the spread of HIV by a wide variety of procedures directed at intravenous drug users, with no one program by itself uniformly effective in preventing HIV transmission. Some countries have embarked on large public education campaigns to teach the means by which HIV is transmitted. Asian governments such as Hong Kong, Malaysia, Singapore, and Thailand have committed extensive financial resources, and specifically, Malaysia and Thailand have undertaken aggressive HIV educational campaigns.

The preliminary results in those two countries have indicated that HIV is not spreading as fast in those areas, compared with the Philippines and Indonesia. Whether the educational campaigns are mainly responsible for this effect is difficult to determine, because other factors such a later onset of HIV, lack of adequate information or changes in behavior, may also be responsible for the slowing of the epidemic. The effectiveness of any of these campaigns is difficult to estimate with a high degree of accuracy.

99. How is AIDS tracked in underdeveloped countries?

Most developing countries lack the means to screen large numbers of people for presence of antibodies against HIV, although there have been increased efforts to bring to developing countries more effective screening tools. In spite of these increased efforts, HIV-antibody tests often cost one dollar a piece, and many countries are unable to afford widespread testing. In the absence of widely accessible HIV-antibody testing sites, asymptomatic carriers go undetected and it becomes difficult to estimate the rate of HIV infection in these countries. Because most AIDS cases are associated with symptoms that are readily observed by health care workers even in areas without sophisticated diagnostic equipment, AIDS cases can be recognized on the basis of the appearance of characteristic symptoms.

The WHO implemented a definition for use in countries without access to HIV-antibody tests or other diagnostic facilities. The definition is intended for use in the field and relies entirely on the presence of symptoms characteristic of AIDS in developing countries. The definition differs slightly for children and adults, and is as follows:

ADULTS

AIDS in an adult is defined by the existence of at least two of the following major signs associated with at least one major sign, in the absence of known causes of immunosuppression such as cancer or preexisting severe malnutrition.

Major Signs
- Weight loss for greater than one month
- Chronic diarrhea for greater than one month
- Prolonged fever for greater than one month, either intermittent or constant

Minor Signs
- Persistent cough for greater than one month
- Generalized itching and inflammation of the skin
- Recurrent herpes zoster
- Candidiasis of the mouth or throat
- Chronic progressive and widespread infection with herpes simplex virus
- Generalized lymphadenopathy

CHILDREN

Pediatric AIDS is suspected in an infant or child presenting with at least two major signs in association with at least two minor signs, in the absence of known causes of immuno-suppression.

Major Signs
- Weight loss or abnormally slow growth
- Chronic diarrhea for greater than one month
- Prolonged fever for greater than one month, intermittent or constant

Minor Signs
- Generalized lymphadenopathy
- Candidiasis of the mouth or throat
- Repeated common infections of the middle ear or mouth
- Persistent cough for greater than one month

- Generalized inflammation of the skin
- Confirmed infection of mother with HIV

The presence of Kaposi's sarcoma or cryptococcal meningitis is sufficient by itself for a person to be diagnosed with AIDS.

100. What is the status of AIDS in Africa?

Cases of AIDS were first noted in Africans seeking treatment in Europe only shortly after AIDS was recognized in the United States. Subsequent epidemiological studies found that AIDS was widespread throughout central Africa with most cases linked by heterosexual contact. Testing of stored blood documented HIV in Africa as early as 1965 and reviews of medical records found cases consistent with AIDS in Africans as early as 1975. A sample of stored blood collected in Africa in 1959 contained HIV, making it the oldest known isolate of the virus. All of these findings indicate that HIV was probably spreading through parts of Africa before it arrived in the United States and in Europe.

It is difficult to determine the true scale of the AIDS epidemic in Africa. Diagnoses are made in only the most obvious cases because of the cost and lack of sophisticated diagnostic equipment. In many parts of Africa, the organized health care delivery system may encounter only a fraction of all AIDS cases. Even in the absence of precise information, Africa holds 15 countries with the highest prevalence of HIV infection in the world. The WHO estimates that more than 13 million Africans are infected with HIV.

HIV infection and AIDS currently account for more than 50% of adult medical admissions and 10% to 15% of pediatric admissions into many national and provincial African hospitals. AIDS is currently the most common cause of death among those aged 15 to 45 years. Greater than 75% of HIV infection in east Africa, where the prevalence of HIV infection is the highest, is transmitted through heterosexual intercourse with an estimated

10% of cases transmitted perinatally. In South Africa, it is estimated that 15% of women of child-bearing age are now infected with HIV.

In some respects the African experience can serve as a model for the United States. The transmissibility of HIV by heterosexual means has been amply demonstrated in Africa. The increase of AIDS in Africa is duplicated in Southeast Asia and is now occurring in India where the prevalence of the virus is growing very rapidly. In each of these cases, the commercial sex industry and the use of drugs have served as potent catalysts to spread HIV throughout a large portion of the heterosexual community. This experience may well be reproduced in the United States, particularly in inner cities. The widespread use of drugs and prostitution, as well as early and frequent sexual activity with many partners, replicate many of the circumstances seen in underdeveloped countries.

101. What is the Haitian link to AIDS?

Early in the epidemic, the high incidence of AIDS in Haitians living in the United States and in parts of Haiti puzzled clinicians. Haitians were first thought to comprise a group at special risk for HIV infection. A variety of theories proposed by some scientists attempted to implicate Haitians in the introduction of HIV infection to the United States. Additional study of HIV infection in Haiti found that the pattern of infection there closely paralleled that found in the heterosexual population of the United States. Although the high incidence of AIDS in Haiti seemed to hold leads for the origin of AIDS, the opposite circumstances seemed more plausible. Instead of Haitians introducing HIV infection into the United States, it is more likely that vacationing Americans or Haitians returning from work in Central Africa had carried HIV to Haiti.

The clustering of AIDS cases around the Carrefour district of Port-au-Prince, the major locale for male and female prostitution in Haiti, supported well-characterized risk factors as the explanation for HIV infection in Haiti. As the epidemic spread further in Haiti, the mode of transmission of HIV remained tightly associated with heterosexual contact. As is the case in Africa, the number of infected females in Haiti nearly equals the number of infected males.

102. Is HIV infection a major problem in prisons?

Prisoners have a high prevalence of HIV infection and AIDS. HIV infection rates are difficult to determine accurately in prison populations because of the high turnover in these groups. For example, local jails may change their inmate population 10 times during the course of a year whereas state facilities have been estimated to turn over their populations about 1.5 times per year. In the United States, the rate of seropositivity in prisons is much higher than the incidence in the general population, even after adjusting for the shifting population.

Estimates calculated in 1996 revealed that by the end of 1994, at least 4588 adult inmates of prisons and jails in the United States died as the result of AIDS, and during 1994, over 5000 adult inmates with AIDS were incarcerated. This latter figure represents 5.2 AIDS cases per 1000 inmates—a rate almost six times that of the total U.S. adult population. Based on the testing of new inmates, HIV seroprevalence rates have varied widely, but have been as high as 22%. Equally alarming is the growing number of confined juveniles with HIV infection. European and some South American prisons also report high seropositivity rates that vary widely from country to country.

Intravenous drug use before incarceration is the most common route of HIV infection in inmates. Unlike the early years of the HIV epidemic in the United States and Europe, where sexual transmission of HIV predominated, intravenous drug use is the predominant risk behavior for HIV infection in prisons. Once in prison, HIV transmission increases through widespread intravenous drug use and homosexual activity. Some studies report that up to 25% of inmates engage in intravenous drug use in prison and that self-reported homosexual activity may range well over 20%. The entry of new inmates to prisons, coupled with HIV infection in already incarcerated individuals, and the prevalence of risky behaviors practiced by them, make prisons a prime location for the spread of HIV. Infected inmates released from prison reenter society carrying HIV and serve as an additional gateway from which HIV is spread into both the homosexual and heterosexual population.

As a result of the high rate of HIV infection in prisoners, some prisons have instituted various policies for inmates. Some United States correctional facilities now provide HIV-antibody testing and both educational materials and risk-reduction counseling to inmates. Testing for HIV antibody is mandatory in some state, city, and county prisons; other prisons test for HIV only when inmates appear to be at high risk for HIV infection or when otherwise medically warranted. Outside the United States, policies for mandatory screening and segregation of HIV-infected inmates differ from country to country.

103. What are the future prospects for HIV infection in the United States?

In many respects the future of AIDS is determined by the past. Those with AIDS today were first infected a median of ten years ago. Those individuals infected today will make up the changing epidemiology and characteristics of future patients with AIDS.

At present, the CDC estimates that between 1 to 1.5 million Americans are infected with HIV. By 1992, HIV infection became the leading cause of death among persons 25 to 44 years of age (Figure 6-4). By 1994, HIV infection remained the leading cause of death in U.S. men and became the third leading cause

Figure 6-4: Death rates* from leading causes of death among men aged 25-44 years, by year — United States, 1982-1994† (From: Centers for Disease Control and Prevention, *Morbidity and Mortality Weekly Report* 1996 45:121-124.)

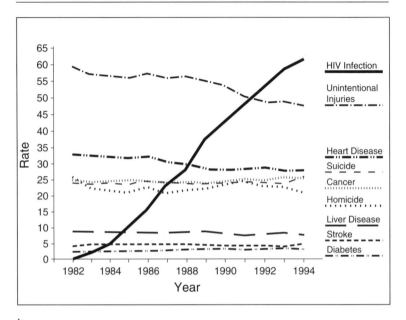

*Per 100,000 population
†National vital statistics based on underlying cause of death, using final data for 1982-1992 and provisional data for 1993-1994.

of death in U.S. women 25 to 44 years of age (Figure 6-5). While improved treatments are assisting people with HIV to live longer, projections by the CDC estimate that by the year 2000, HIV will become the leading cause of death among Americans.

The HIV-AIDS epidemic is composed of several smaller epidemics in different populations. During the 1990s, Blacks have had a greater proportional increase in rates of HIV infection as compared with Whites. This is reflected in death rates from AIDS (Figure 6-6). Similarly, the rate of persons with AIDS infected through heterosexual contact is greater compared with those acquiring AIDS by other transmission modes. Over 2% of the

Figure 6-5: Death rates* from leading causes of death among women aged 25-44 years, by year — United States, 1982-1994† (From: Centers for Disease Control and Prevention, *Morbidity and Mortality Weekly Report* 1996, 45:121-124.)

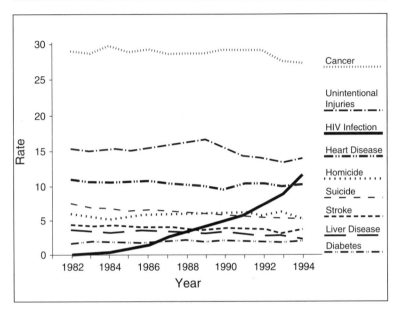

*Per 100,000 population.
†National vital statistics based on underlying cause of death, using final data for 1982-1992 and provisional data for 1993-1994.

nearly 1 million prisoners incarcerated in United States prisons are infected with HIV, a rate 7 times greater than the general population. Women of childbearing age constitute a growing population of HIV-infected persons, and perinatal transmission of HIV is increasing at an alarming rate. In addition, the increasing death rate from AIDS for women (Figure 6-5), who acquire HIV infection primarily through sexual contact with injecting drug-using partners, affects the care of their children: it has been estimated that among 80,000 HIV-infected women of child-bearing age who were alive in 1992, more than 100,000 children will be orphaned when their infected mothers die during this decade.

Figure 6-6: Death rates˙ from HIV infection among persons aged 25-44 years, by sex, race§, and year — United States, 1982-1994† (§Data were unavailable for races other than white and black.) (From: Centers for Disease Control and Prevention, *Morbidity and Mortality Weekly Report* 1996, 45:121-124.)

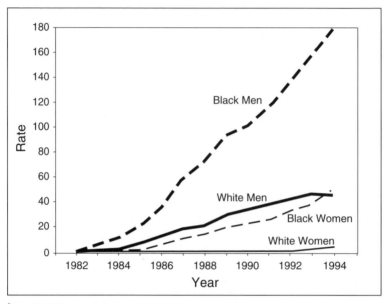

˙Per 100,000 population.
†National vital statistics based on underlying cause of death, using final data for 1982-1992 and provisional data for 1993-1994.

Just as prior HIV infection over the last decade reflects current AIDS trends, current HIV infections will alter the changing demographics of AIDS within the next decade. As importantly, information on HIV-related mortality within the next decade will allow an appreciation of the effectiveness of current therapies and education programs.

104. What are the projected costs of AIDS in the United States?

The cost of AIDS is measured in many different forms. Years of life lost, medical expenses, lost productivity, and human suffering all demonstrate the same fact: AIDS is costly in every respect. In 1992, AIDS became and has remained the leading cause of death among men in the United States between the ages of 25 and 45. AIDS is currently the third leading cause of death for women in the same age range. The effect of early deaths on overall longevity is estimated by years of potential life lost, a measure of premature deaths occurring before 65 years of age. AIDS is now the leading cause of potential life lost in the United States among males aged 15 to 64 years, surpassing homicides, suicides, heart disease, and cancer.

During 1995, the number of reported AIDS cases in the United States was 55,573. With a conservative estimate of the total lifetime costs of HIV infection and AIDS at $95,000, the estimated 50-60,000 new American AIDS cases in 1996 will cost over 5 billion dollars for health care and supportive services.

In the absence of any new infections, a significant number of the 1.5 million Americans currently infected with HIV will develop AIDS in the next ten years. These anticipated AIDS cases and deaths will likely exceed the cumulative 566,000 American deaths in World Wars I and II, the Korean War, and the Vietnam War.

AIDS deaths in young women are leaving a tragic legacy: AIDS orphans. Conservative estimates project that in the United States, more than 35,000 children and adolescents will be left motherless by 1997—those projections could total over 100,000 orphans by the year 2000. Disrupted family structures and frequent poverty put these AIDS orphans at increased risk for a variety of social ills, including AIDS. Limited formal support mechanisms exist for these children who will grow in number and expand the already increasing demands on the social services in large and small cities. Data that describe the size of this problem in underdeveloped countries are lacking. Africa,

Southeast Asia, and South America already face an onslaught of children orphaned by AIDS who have very limited recourse to address their most basic domestic, educational, and health needs.

—CHAPTER SEVEN—

Treatment of HIV Infection

105. What is the basis for developing drugs active against infections?

Successful treatments for infections of any kind, whether fungal, bacterial, or viral, exploit biological differences between the offending microorganism and the infected host or cell. A well-known example is penicillin. It is a product of a common mold and is toxic to some types of bacteria that frequently cause disease in humans. The key to the success of this antibiotic is that it is toxic to bacteria but not toxic to humans. It is selective toxicity that kills or renders harmless an infecting microorganism while simultaneously allowing a drug to be given to humans without harm or with limited, but acceptable, side effects.

Effective drugs interfere with chemical processes that are essential to the infecting microorganism. Microorganisms with their own set of metabolic processes that differ from human processes often provide attractive targets for therapy. The best targets for therapy are the unique proteins supplied by the infecting organism and not present in the host. Organisms with few unique chemical processes have few acceptable targets for drugs. Because HIV provides only very few proteins of its own for its growth and reproduction, it has a very limited number of potential chemical targets for inhibition. Although many different proteins are necessary for the reproduction of HIV, all of the additional proteins not carried by the virus are supplied by the infected host cell. Because these additional proteins are of cellular origin, interfering with their function may be highly detrimental to the cell and cause unacceptable side effects in the treated patient.

106. What are the therapeutic approaches used to treat HIV infection?

A variety of different drugs active against HIV exist. Most of the agents with demonstrated clinical utility act directly on the virus. These drugs can be understood by grouping them with the different stages of the HIV life cycle that they attempt to inhibit. Potent inhibitors directed against some of the essential steps of HIV replication slow viral growth and result in an improved clinical outcome for patients receiving those therapies. Other approaches use a strategy called immune-based therapy, but there is little evidence that the strategies employed to date are useful in the treatment of HIV infection. New lines of investigation may identify immune-based approaches with some usefulness, but these strategies have no immediate role in the treatment of HIV infection outside research programs.

The first step in HIV reproduction is attachment of the virus to the host cell and entry of the virus into the cell (Figure 7-1). Agents that interfere with the binding and entry of HIV to cells have been identified but were ineffective in all studies. Early approaches used soluble CD4 molecules to mimic the natural receptor for HIV and bind HIV before it encountered cells susceptible to infection. Use of this agent failed to produce useful virologic activity in clinical trials. Other approaches that exploit a newly identified molecule on the surface of lymphocytes called fusin may yield new drugs, but no drugs that inhibit fusin exist at this time.

The next useful drug target is reverse transcription. This step requires the enzyme reverse transcriptase which is provided by HIV. Reverse transcriptase transcribes, or copies, viral RNA into DNA that is then introduced into the DNA of the host cell. Because this is essential to HIV reproduction, reverse transcription is a particularly attractive target for drugs. Agents that inhibit reverse transcriptase benefit infected humans. Zidovudine (ZDV or AZT), didanosine (ddI), zalcitabine (ddC), lamivudine (3TC), and stavudine (D4T) are the most common reverse transcriptase

Figure 7-1: Antiviral agents may inhibit any of several steps in the HIV life cycle: 1) attachment to host cell membrane, 2) reverse transcription of viral RNA to DNA, 3) transcription of viral cDNA integrated into host cell DNA, or 4) translation and assembly of viral RNA and proteins. Notably, reverse transcription is inhibited by agents such as zidovudine, and translation of viral RNA and proteins is inhibited by agents such as indinavir and ritonavir. (From: *AIDS: Problems and Prospects*, by Lawrence Corey, M.D., editor. Copyright ©1993, 1992, 1991, 1990 by HP Publishing Co., New York, NY. Reprinted by permission of W.W. Norton & Company, Inc.)

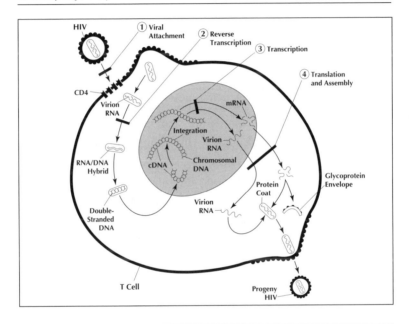

inhibitors used to treat patients with HIV infection. After reverse transcription, viral RNA is copied into DNA. This viral DNA must be introduced into cellular DNA by the virally encoded integrase enzyme. No drugs tested in humans inhibit this important process in HIV, although some pharmaceutical companies are pursuing this approach as a strategy to inhibit HIV growth.

Steps subsequent to reverse transcription and integration of DNA produce new, intact viruses that emerge from the infected cell. Most of these steps rely on cellular proteins and not on viral proteins. The lack of steps using viral proteins makes identifying agents with selective activity very difficult. One viral target called HIV protease is particularly attractive for the treatment of HIV infection. HIV protease is an enzyme that is essential for viral reproduction; if it is absent or inhibited, virus is unable to grow. HIV protease is uniquely responsible for completing the processing of the virus from an immature form that is not infectious, into a mature form that readily infects susceptible cells. Protease is active as the immature HIV particle emerges from the surface of the cell in which it is produced. As HIV passes through the membrane, HIV protease carries out its function which leads to a mature, infectious particle that is released from the cell that made it. Inhibiting this enzyme allows for the production of viral particles, however, they are unable to infect new cells. Sufficiently long inhibition of this enzyme will allow infected cells to die without being replaced by a newly infected cell. Over a matter of days to weeks, the majority of infected cells die leading to large reductions in viral titers with the agents that are potent and tested to date. Protease inhibitors that are useful in the treatment of HIV infection are indinavir, ritonavir, saquinavir, and nelfinavir.

Physicians use these drugs in many different combinations. Clinical trial data indicate that the combined use of these agents—often combining protease inhibitors with reverse transcriptase inhibitors—is nearly always superior to use of any one drug by itself. Drugs with similar resistance patterns, or other metabolic considerations that interfere with drug elimination from the body, or unacceptable side effects, should not be combined. Usually regimens are structured to achieve maximal reductions in viral RNA. To do so, most regimens contain at least one very potent agent that is likely to produce large declines in viral titers.

107. What are the therapeutic options for persons infected with HIV?

At this writing, several drugs are available for the treatment of HIV infection in the United States and in many other countries. These drugs fall into two broad classes, reverse transcriptase inhibitors and protease inhibitors. The reverse transcriptase inhibitors include zidovudine (ZDV, also known as AZT), zalcitabine (ddC), didanosine (ddI), lamivudine (3TC), stavudine (d4T), and nevirapine. All of the reverse transcriptase inhibitors, except nevirapine, are called nucleoside analogues because of their chemical relatedness to the building blocks of DNA, the nucleosides. Despite their chemical similarities to each other and nearly indistinguishable abilities to lower the level of HIV in the bloodstream, each nucleoside analogue has unique side effects which often dictate how they are used. Nevirapine is also a reverse transcriptase inhibitor, but it is not a nucleoside analogue.

All of the licensed nucleoside reverse transcriptase inhibitors cause side effects that can range from troublesome to dangerous. While 3TC is relatively well tolerated, ZDV routinely decreases blood cell production often resulting in anemia or newtropenia. This toxicity may require either stopping the drug, reducing the amount of ZDV administered, or adding specific therapies (e.g., colony-stimulating factors) to increase blood cell counts to normal ranges. Some patients also experience headache, stomach upset, and a gradual wasting of muscles beyond that expected with AIDS alone. Although d4T, ddI, and ddC do not cause blood abnormalities, they can damage peripheral nerves, leading to a condition called neuropathy. These drugs can affect the longest nerves in the body involving sensation and produce a neuropathy manifested by painful sensations called paresthesias. Stopping the drug sufficiently early after the appearance of symptoms usually reverses the paresthesias. A potentially life-threatening side effect called pancreatitis, inflammation of the pancreas, affects some patients receiving ddI. Careful monitoring of patients receiving this drug and avoiding other medications that can cause pancreatitis, including alcohol, limits the likelihood of developing this side effect. Nevirapine use can be associated with a rash which infrequently is dangerous. Frequent and sometimes severe side effects for these drugs must be weighed against the consequences of not treating HIV infection; the risk-benefit balance favors therapy with these drugs in most cases.

Another class of compounds called protease inhibitors also is used to treat HIV infection. Three protease inhibitors are approved and others are expected to follow. The approved compounds are indinavir, ritonavir, and saquinavir. Nelfinavir is expected to be the fourth protease inhibitor approved in the United States. These compounds are chemically related, but they are differentiated from each other by their activity and by their ease of administration to patients. Saquinavir is well-tolerated by patients but has low antiretroviral activity. Indinavir requires strict dietary regimentation and often causes kidney stones, while ritonavir frequently produces nausea. However, both indinavir and ritonavir have profound antiviral activity.

108. What is the most desirable treatment for HIV infection?

Clinical and epidemiological studies unequivocally find that individuals who have low levels of HIV in blood, either with or without therapy, live longer and have fewer HIV-related complications than patients who have higher levels of virus. Potent antiretroviral agents that inhibit HIV at various points in its lifecycle can now routinely reduce levels of HIV to very low, and sometimes undetectable levels. Although the full duration of the antiviral activity is unknown, the therapeutic benefits can be substantial. A consensus is emerging that the goal of therapy is to reduce HIV to the lowest possible levels through the use of antiretroviral drugs and to maintain it at those levels as long as possible.

Although a vast number of clinical trials are complete and others underway, it is impossible to identify a single best regimen for all patients. Instead, it is clear that multiple different regimens exist that now promise substantial clinical benefits. Physicians should plan therapeutic regimens with their patients in a way that considers drugs the patients have already received, the antiretroviral activity of combined agents, the toxicity of the regimen, and the ability of the patient to comply with the prescribed drug regimen.

Ultimately, the most ambitious goal of any HIV therapy is ridding the body of the virus. This is complicated by the integration of HIV into the genetic material of the host cell. The basic strategy employed by current drug regimens reduces the level of virus by relying on the natural cell death of infected cells. This death, when not matched by the infection of a replacement cell, gradually lowers the total number of infected cells in the body that are producing HIV and thereby results in lower levels of HIV in the blood. A tantalizing question in HIV therapeutics concerns the duration of highly suppressive therapy necessary to exceed the lifespan of the longest-lived infected cell in the body. If it is possible for the last HIV-infected cell to die, then HIV will have been eradicated from the body. Scientists anxiously await a first report of viral eradication. While theoretically possible, no detailed estimates of the duration of highly suppressive therapy necessary for viral eradication exist. Patients embarking upon antiretroviral therapy, therefore, should assume that their treatment will be lifelong.

109. Is it possible to regenerate the immune system?

The hallmark of HIV infection is progressive loss of a set of T lymphocytes, the CD4 cells. Although the precise means by which these cells die remain elusive, their loss results in profound immune compromise. Many immunological abnormalities exist in persons with AIDS, most of which are related to CD4 cell function. Some of the important abnormalities include nonspecific activation of antibody-producing cells (B lymphocytes), altered levels of the antiviral protein interferon, and decreased immune activity of other types of lymphocytes. It would seem, therefore, that transfusing CD4 cells into an AIDS patient would contribute much to the reconstitution of the immune system. Isolated CD4 cells, however, are difficult to obtain in large numbers and are usually incompatible with the resident cells of a prospective recipient. Physicians have attempted, therefore, to replace some of the factors produced by an activated immune system. Interferon, interleukin-2, and tumor necrosis factor are some of the compounds generated by the immune system. Studies fail to demonstrate that these compounds reconstitute the immune system or improve the clinical course of patients suffering from AIDS.

A more radical approach to treating the defective immune system is to replace it. Because the bone marrow produces lymphocytes, the most aggressive approach to reconstitute the immune system is to transplant a healthy bone marrow into an infected patient. This procedure has yielded only very transient benefits in the few patients who received it. The failure of even bone marrow transplantation illustrates the difficulty of replacing lymphocytes in patients infected with HIV. Almost certainly the patients continue to harbor the virus elsewhere in the body and then reinfect the donated lymphocytes. Replacing lymphocytes by themselves is thus not a viable therapeutic option. The development of new, highly effective antiretroviral regimens raises the possibility of identifying new therapies or approaches to regenerating the immune system. Use of protease inhibitor therapy combined with other drugs has produced limited reconstitution of immunity in some patients.

110. What is the evidence that antiretroviral therapy benefits patients?

Agents that are active against HIV have observable antiretroviral activity within seven days of initiating the drug. This activity is readily seen using HIV PCR and bDNA viral monitoring techniques. There is a gradient of antiretroviral activity with different agents used either as monotherapy or in combination. Most nucleoside agents reach maximal declines in viral RNA of around 50% to 60%. When multiple nucleosides are combined, declines in excess of 90% to 95% can occur, especially if the patient is receiving both drugs for the first time. Protease inhibitors often achieve 99% to 99.9% declines in viral titers for a limited period of time. When drugs are combined, especially a protease inhibitor with one or two nucleosides, patients sustain viral titer reductions beyond 99% for months, and perhaps years. The maximal duration of therapy when used in this manner is unknown. Combination use of a drug can be influenced by prior exposure to the agent, especially if for many weeks. Previous exposure to a drug in a therapeutic regimen may blunt the subsequent activity of the already administered drug, even when used in combination, because of the rapid development of viral resistance.

A variety of clinical trials using antiretroviral therapy either based on nucleosides or using protease inhibitors produced data that are useful for verifying the clinical benefit of this approach to treatment. Studies find that a two-fold reduction in viral titers produces a 27% decrement in the risk for HIV disease progression. A three-fold effect in another study found a 63% reduction in the risk of disease progression, and a 90% lowering of viral titers produced an 80% decrement in the risk of disease progression. The goal of therapy, therefore, is the maximal possible reduction in viral titers, via whatever regimen achieves that reduction, for as long as possible. Despite frequent references to triple and more complicated drug cocktails in the lay press, no data establish the superiority of any triple drug regimen to any other less complicated regimen when similar viral titer declines are attained.

111. How do physicians decide to initiate antiretroviral therapy?

A variety of opinions exist on the proper point to initiate anti-retroviral therapy. Recent clinical trial data established a clear link between clinical outcomes and viral titer reductions in patients receiving therapy. In addition, natural history data unambiguously find that worsening prognoses are tied to higher HIV blood titers. Because the central goal of treating patients with HIV infection is to prevent disease progression and death, many physicians believe that HIV titers should determine the point at which treatment begins. A strict interpretation of this general approach holds that as soon as a patient is identified with HIV infection, treatment should be initiated. Provided that the treatment goals are achievable, this approach makes sense. On the other hand, the duration of therapy may be lifelong in patients with HIV infection and any delay in the initiation of therapy, provided patients do not deteriorate in a clinically significant way, avoids potentially unnecessary and expensive therapy. In addition, treatment can provide virus with an opportunity to become resistant to therapy. If patients do not properly comply with their regimen and resistance develops, patients may lose the opportunity for substantial clinical benefit from the drugs in the failed regimen.

Because of the counterbalancing issues of disease progression and the risk of therapeutic failure, some physicians believe that treatment should be initiated when HIV titers are greater than 30,000 copies of HIV RNA per mL of blood. For patients with lower titers, the patient's CD4 cell count also should be consi-dered in determining the urgency of beginning treatment. The goal of therapy is to reach viral titers that are as low as possible. Assuming that the natural history data relating outcomes to viral titers will match the outcomes achieved when patients reach those same titers on therapy, fewer than 5,000 copies of HIV RNA per mL is viewed as an attractive target. However, information relating outcomes on therapy to specific average HIV RNA levels does not exist.

There are no rigid rules in the treatment of HIV infection. All guidelines are recommendations that are subject to interpretation on an individualized basis. Although not formalized by HIV RNA levels or CD4 cell counts, once a patient develops an AIDS-defining illness regardless of the CD4 cell level, most patients will benefit from antiretroviral therapy at that point. All physicians must carefully assess the ability of a patient to comply with any regimen prescribed to determine if a desired therapeutic outcome is likely. Data from clinical studies usually describes average responses for a large number of patients; physicians, however, must care for patients on an individual basis.

112. What is the role of PCR and bDNA in the treatment of HIV infection?

Both PCR and bDNA are very sensitive and reproducible techniques used to measure the level of HIV RNA present in body fluids. Because individual HIV particles contain RNA—the material in which HIV carries its genetic information—measurement of viral RNA can be used to determine the number of HIV particles in a clinical sample. Although both PCR and bDNA are typically used to measure the level of HIV in the blood, researchers are attempting to extend use of these techniques to detect HIV in other body fluids and tissues.

The development of PCR and bDNA led to important insights into how the HIV virus causes disease and how to treat HIV infection with antiretroviral therapy. The accurate measurement of viral levels in blood has revealed that the amount of HIV produced every day is much greater than previously thought: between 1 billion and 10 billion HIV particles are generated daily in the body from cells infected with HIV. In addition, higher numbers of HIV particles are present in the blood of people with advanced HIV disease compared with people at earlier stages of HIV disease.

The detection of high levels of HIV in all stages of the disease, and the correlation between high viral levels and worsening prognosis, provided key insights that led to significant improvements in HIV therapeutics. For example, large numbers of HIV particles produced each day explained the rapid development of viral resistance to many antiretroviral therapies. The greater the number of particles produced each day, the greater the chances that random changes or mutations in the molecular structure of HIV will produce particles resistant to a drug regimen. The enormous production of HIV also accounted for the loss of CD4 lymphocytes over the course of HIV infection. Viral particles kill CD4 lymphocytes and trigger other immunological responses that further reduce the number of lymphocytes. Humans produce a vast number of lymphocytes during their lifetime, but it appears that the numbers of HIV particles produced and CD4 lymphocytes destroyed exceed the capacity of the body to produce lymphocytes. This process culminates in an ever lower number of lymphocytes and decreasing immunological function that ultimately results in the clinical manifestations of HIV infection.

The link between HIV levels and prognosis is that lower levels of virus predict a better prognosis than higher levels of virus. Furthermore, drugs with activity against HIV produce readily detected changes in viral levels in the blood. For example, triple-drug regimens containing a protease inhibitor and two reverse transcriptase inhibitors often result in very low levels of HIV RNA as detected by PCR and bDNA. Scientists also have found other regimens with similar antiretroviral activity. Thus, PCR and bDNA have become vital tools in the treatment of HIV infection. The goal of therapy is the maximal reduction of HIV levels in blood for the longest possible time. Showing an initial reduction in virus levels after initiating drug treatment is not adequate evidence that a patient will continue to benefit from such therapy. If the virus continues to grow in the body, even at low levels, HIV mutants that are resistant to the administered drug may be produced. Virus growth at high levels during therapy warrants modification of the antiretroviral regimen because of the significant likelihood of resistance to and decreased therapeutic efficacy of the drug regimen. Thus, the only way to determine whether a given drug regimen continues to produce the desired effect on viral titers is the periodic assessment of blood viral levels while on therapy.

Techniques to measure viral RNA levels are increasingly available to physicians who care for persons with HIV infection. As the sensitivity of these tests increases, physicians will be able to design drug regimens that decrease virus amounts to even lower levels than presently achievable. Terms such as "undetectable virus" do not mean that HIV is not present in a sample of blood or body tissue. Instead, this term means that the level of virus has decreased to levels below which current assay techniques accurately can detect. PCR and bDNA have lower levels of detection that range from 200 to 500 HIV particles per ml of blood, levels that are well below those observed in most patients before they begin antiretroviral therapy. However, these low levels, once achieved with therapy, still permit sufficient virus growth to generate HIV mutants resistant to therapy. Only improvements in drug development and technologies that better determine viral load will permit better management of patients and optimize therapeutic regimens.

113. What is the life expectancy of patients who receive zidovudine therapy?

Although several different drugs are licensed in the United States to treat HIV infection, much more survival information is known about ZDV than any of the other drugs. A study in the United States retrospectively examined through a systematic review of medical records the course of patients receiving ZDV shortly after the drug became available in the United States in 1987 and 1988. Patients were selected if at the time of starting the study they had a CD4 count at or below 250 and either had AIDS, including at least one previous infection with *Pneumocystis carinii*, or AIDS-related complex as originally defined by the CDC.

The median survival of patients was determined in part by the CD4 cell count at the time when ZDV was begun at entry to the study. Patients with an initial CD4 count of greater than or equal to 150/μL had a median survival of over 900 days. After one year of ZDV therapy, survival was 90%, decreasing to 56% after 2.5 years of ZDV therapy. Patients who began ZDV therapy with low CD4 counts had a short median survival. The median survival for patients with initial CD4 counts less than 50/μL was 560 days with 75% of the patients surviving one year and 19% surviving 2.5 years. Patients who began the study with ARC had rates of progression to AIDS that were influenced by initial CD4 cell counts. The median time to progression to AIDS in patients with ARC and a CD4 count greater than or equal to 150/μL was 810 days; this decreased to 310 days for patients with CD4 cell counts below 50/μL. There is no evidence that African-Americans, Hispanics, women, or intravenous drug users have different responses to therapy than those indicated here.

This study began in the late 1980s and may not be entirely representative of patients who initiated therapy with ZDV at later dates. The standard of care of AIDS patients is continually improving, new therapies exist that were not available to many patients who participated in this study, and prophylaxis for PCP is now common practice although not widely used when the study began. The results of this study, when compared with historical data accumulated before retroviral therapy, indicate that ZDV greatly improved the prognosis of patients with AIDS and ARC. The prognosis for patients developing AIDS in the 1990s may be better than these figures because of identification of new drugs active against HIV and the attendant opportunistic infections. General considerations already discussed document the survival advantage of patients treated with effective therapy. The true survival of patients who use currently available therapy that maximally suppresses HIV RNA blood titers and sustains that reduction is not known. There is little reason to believe that patients who gain deep and sustained HIV titer reductions at a point sufficiently early in their disease will not have profound improvements in both the morbidity and mortality historically associated with AIDS.

114. Does HIV develop resistance to antiviral drugs?

Resistance of HIV to antiviral compounds does occur and has several implications. As HIV becomes resistant to drugs, the beneficial effect of the drug will be diminished or lost entirely. The loss of therapeutic effect has obvious negative consequences for an individual receiving the drug, but with time it is possible that resistant viruses will also spread through the general population, gradually rendering the drug useless. HIV recovered from untreated patients is currently nearly uniformly sensitive to most new drugs, making the possible widespread presence of resistant HIV a hypothetical concern. However, ZDV resistance in HIV-infected individuals never previously treated with the drug is an expanding problem.

Studies have demonstrated that, although most isolates of HIV obtained from patients are sensitive to ZDV before its administration, resistance develops rapidly in some groups of patients who receive ZDV for prolonged periods. Physicians following patients receiving ZDV for many months found that the likelihood of detecting resistant virus was both a function of length of therapy and the CD4 cell count of the patient. One report found that, for patients with CD4 counts less than 100 at the initiation of therapy, resistance developed at a rate of 63% to 99% after one year of treatment. For patients with CD4 cells from 100 to 400 and for those with greater than 400 CD4 cells, the rate of resistance at one year of therapy was 18% to 75% and 11% to 59%, respectively. The prognostic significance of resistance is incompletely defined for patients with resistant strains of virus, although a loss of virus suppression while receiving therapy generally limits the therapeutic utility of continued treatment with the drug.

As the clinical experience with all drugs active against HIV grows, viral resistance to these drugs increasingly is observed. Only additional observation with these drugs will define the occurrence of resistance and if such resistance will limit the use of the drugs. Clinical research indicates that combining anti-retroviral drugs appropriately minimizes the occurrence of resistence.

115. Does any therapy prevent infection in individuals recently exposed to HIV?

There are limited circumstances in which therapy is known to prevent infection after an acute exposure to HIV: prevention of HIV transmission from woman to child and to a person pierced with an HIV-contaminated needle. The use of ZDV to interrupt the spread of HIV during pregnancy is perhaps one of the most important therapeutic developments during the HIV epidemic. Cases of HIV infection are prevented by this practice and done so in a highly cost-effective manner. Use of this drug reduces the risk of transmission from about 25% in persons not receiving treatment to about 8% in women receiving the drug. Infants born to infected women typically receive some therapy for a limited period after birth with ZDV in the treatment regimen used in this study. Although the use of ZDV in pregnancy is very effective, efforts are underway to improve on the already low rate of transmission in pregnancy. Cesarean section to date has not been shown to be an effective measure in reducing the transmission of HIV to infants.

Already approved drugs, especially ZDV, have been examined for activity in preventing infection after a person has been accidentally stuck with a needle containing HIV-contaminated blood. The low rate of seroconversion from this type of exposure makes accumulating enough patients to answer this question with precision difficult. Nonetheless, many hospitals provided ZDV at standard doses for several weeks after accidental exposure to

HIV-contaminated blood by needlestick or other penetrating injuries. The value of this practice was established by a large case-control study that found that treatment with ZDV after a needlestick or similar percutaneous injury reduced the risk of infection by almost 80%. New recommendations from the CDC for post-exposure prophylaxis (PEP) suggest the use of two nucleosides (zidovudine and lamivudine) along with a protease inhibitor, preferably begun within one to two hours after exposure and taken for four weeks. No data exist that describes at which point after exposure PEP ceases to protect against infection but recommendations have been made to begin therapy as soon as possible, especially within 24 to 36 hours after known or possible exposure to HIV. Physicians may wish to tailor the drugs used in PEP on a case-by-case basis when sufficient information exists on the source of the exposure to guide selection of agents that may be more appropriate than those recommended by the CDC. In addition, benefits of initiating therapy after the interval thought to be effective (24 to 36 hours after exposure) are not defined and should be evaluated on an individual basis.

The same general considerations probably hold for individuals acutely exposed to HIV in occupational exposures by means other than a needlestick, although no circumstance has been as well studied as needlestick PEP. No guidelines exist for sexual exposure to HIV infection. Healthy patients who do receive a short course of the recommended agents after an exposure run little risk of suffering very significant adverse clinical effects from the drugs.

116. Is therapy beneficial in primary HIV infection?

No controlled clinical trial with a sufficient number of patients has been completed to test if ZDV, or any other therapy, confers a meaningful benefit during primary infection with HIV. The logistics of finding adequate numbers of individuals, who must then be followed for years after receiving therapy or placebo, make this study difficult.

Reasons to consider treating with antiretroviral therapy during the primary infection include the possibility of eliminating HIV from the body during an early phase of the illness, mitigating the clinical symptoms of primary infection and altering the long-term consequences of HIV infection. A small pilot study suggested that patients who received ZDV at the onset of the symptoms of the primary infection were able to tolerate therapy for a limited course with minimal side effects. However, these patients all had changes in HIV p24 antigen levels similar to that reported for patients who had not received ZDV and no clear evidence of any reduction in the severity of their initial symptoms. Several patients in this study had virus isolated from their bloodstream after therapy, indicating that ZDV when used very early in the course of HIV infection does not prevent the establishment of HIV in the body. No data were available on the long-term outcome of these patients.

Another small study found that although ZDV therapy did not influence the symptoms during the acute infection, the rate of opportunistic infections in the ensuing months was lower in the treated group than in the placebo group. The long-term consequences of therapy with ZDV at this stage of the infection are unknown. At the present time there is no consensus on the use of ZDV or any antiretroviral regimen in primary HIV infection. There are, however, small numbers of patients treated with ZDV, 3TC, and ritonavir, a protease inhibitor, in which nearly all patients reach extremely low levels of HIV in the blood. Although the clinical consequences of this regimen when used at the earliest stage of infection are unclear, the virological effects are very promising. Studies in progress may provide more information, but it is unlikely for logistical reasons that large-scale trials will ever be completed.

117. To what extent will antiretroviral therapy decrease transmission of HIV from a pregnant woman to her child?

Maternal-infant transmission is the main way in which children become infected with HIV. Pregnancy in an HIV-infected woman carries a 20% to 30% risk of transmission of HIV to an infant. A key study was published in 1994 that showed the effectiveness of zidovudine (ZDV) in reducing this risk.

HIV-infected women who had not received prior ZDV therapy received a regimen of ZDV beginning at 14 to 34 weeks of gestation and continuing throughout pregnancy, including labor and delivery. Additionally, newborns received ZDV therapy for six weeks after birth. At 18 months of age, 8% of the infants in the ZDV group were HIV-infected compared with 25% in the group not receiving ZDV. Subsequent studies have shown a relationship between increased maternal HIV-1 RNA levels (viral load) and increased risk of perinatal transmission. The benefits of ZDV in this setting have resulted in strong recommendations by the United States Public Health Service to encourage HIV education programs and voluntary testing of all pregnant women.

Recent studies have shown the significant challenges that educational programs to reduce the risk of perinatal transmission present. Pregnant, HIV-infected women identified through an urban medical center in the United States and considered candidates for ZDV therapy were contacted. About 75% of women began therapy. Women refusing therapy were more likely to report injecting drug use as their main risk factor for HIV disease, and were also more likely to continue injecting drug use during their pregnancy. Among the women receiving ZDV, approximately one-third did not adhere to their regimen, and this was associated with a significant number of women who continued using cocaine.

Since 1994, several states (e.g., North Carolina and Connecticut) have passed legislation requiring that health care providers notify all pregnant women of the availability of HIV testing.

118. How can one estimate the prognosis of patients?

Physicians follow two types of information in estimating the prognosis of an HIV patient: laboratory indicators and clinical indicators.

The laboratory test with the greatest utility in estimating prognosis are the RNA-based HIV titer techniques, PCR and bDNA. Studies using these techniques find that blood titers generally correlate with the stage of disease; after initial infection when titers are briefly high, patients who remain asymptomatic tend to have lower titers than patients who progress to advanced disease. Individual patients, however, tend to maintain a level of HIV that is relatively constant over time in the absence of therapy. The factors that influence the "set point" HIV titer in any one patient not on antiretroviral therapy are unknown. Prolonged follow-up studies find that more than 70% of patients with CD4 cell counts above 500 cells/μL and with HIV titers in excess of 10,200 progressed to AIDS or death within ten years of their viral titer determination, whereas less than 30% of patients with similar CD4 cell counts but lower viral titers reached those endpoints within the same time period. In particular, 62% of patients with more than 36,270 HIV particles/mL of blood will develop AIDS within five years, assuming that effective therapeutic intervention does not occur. Individuals with between 13,021 and 36,270 particles/mL progress to AIDS in 49% of cases within five years. Individuals with levels between 4530 and 13,020 particles/mL progress to AIDS in 26% of cases within five years. Patients with the lowest levels of virus, those with less than 4531 particles/mL of blood, progress to AIDS in only 8% of the cases within five years.

Survival during HIV infection is also closely linked to the level of virus in the blood. For the same group of patients already described, 49%, 25%, 10%, and 5% of patients died within five years of determination of HIV levels that ranged from high to low, respectively. These studies showed that the CD4 count added little information for estimating the rate of progression to

AIDS or death. This work makes clear the central role of HIV RNA levels in determining the prognosis for an individual patient. Although a limited number of studies have explored the role of reducing HIV levels in response to therapy, in every case a reduction in HIV resulted in a reduced rate of disease progression and, in studies in which survival was examined, improved survival.

CD4 lymphocyte levels, a readily accessible and reasonably reproducible laboratory indicator, provide only a fair estimate of the prognosis for disease progression and survival, but they are more useful in estimating the general risk for opportunistic infections. For example, fewer than 5% of patients will suffer an AIDS-defining illness or death in the 24 months after a CD4 cell determination of greater than 500 cells/µL of blood. This low rate of AIDS complications contrasts with a rate of more than 70% of patients developing HIV disease or death in 24 months in patients with fewer than 50 CD4 cells/µL. Because low CD4 counts often herald the onset of clinically significant disease, physicians traditionally tied the initiation of antiretroviral therapy to CD4 cell levels, although new information makes this practice obsolete. Other laboratory values do add some limited information to CD4 levels. Elevated blood levels of either beta-microglobulin or neopterin, molecules produced by the activated immune system, coupled with low CD4 levels indicate a very high risk of progression to AIDS, but have little use in clinical practice because other techniques provide more information.

Determining the prognosis for HIV-infected persons is an evolving process made difficult by the long interval between symptom-free HIV infection and AIDS. Indeed, although some patients progress to AIDS shortly after documented HIV infection, more than 10% remain symptom-free over 15 years after initial infection. Therapeutic advances made during the lifetime of a patient can render existing prognostic information obsolete. In particular, the prognostic information of the RNA-based assays was collected when protease inhibitors were not available to the patients participating in the prognostic studies.

Patients in whom a viral determination is made who then begin therapy that achieves substantial HIV suppression for a prolonged period will have prognoses that are better than those reported here. In general, the basic principle that HIV titers predict clinical outcomes is established. Therapy is therefore centered on reducing HIV titers as low as possible in patients. As long as new therapies are developed and standards of care raised rapidly, prognostic information will always lag and probably underestimate the true prognosis of a patient beginning treatment for HIV infection.

119. Is the progression of HIV infection influenced by the strain of HIV that has infected the person?

Laboratory studies indicate there may be a relationship between progressing to AIDS and the growth properties of the infecting strain of HIV. Those infected with strains of HIV that grow rapidly when isolated in laboratory culture conditions and cause syncytia, lymphocytes that fuse into clumps, progress to AIDS more rapidly than those with virus that does not cause syncytia or that grows slowly. Evidence that growth properties of HIV can change during infection to increasingly virulent forms is accumulating.

The rate of change of HIV growth patterns varies from person to person. Those with slow-growing HIV have a slow decline in CD4 numbers, whereas people with a virus that grows more quickly and results in a higher viral titer in blood have a more rapid decline in their CD4 cell numbers. A person may initially have a slow-growing virus that becomes a fast-growing one over the course of the infection. Determination of the rate of viral growth and syncytium-inducing qualities of HIV in individual patients is not a routine virological procedure. These tests are research tools and are not used to stage a patient's infection or influence therapy. Another study also suggests that the strain infecting a person may influence the clinical course of his or her disease. A study in Australia found that six infected transfusion recipients from a common donor all remained free of symptoms for an unusually long period of time. Only one patient developed AIDS during an observation period ranging from 6.8 to 10.1 years. This low rate of progression contrasts with other transfusion-related AIDS cases. A total of 94 out of 101 comparable patients developed AIDS or a CD4 cell count less than 50/µL in only a seven year observation period. This study suggests that a weakly pathogenic strain infected both donor and recipients. In general, however, the titer of HIV in the blood is far more predictive of clinical outcomes than determining if the virus is of a particular strain and then attempting to estimate a prognosis for a patient.

120. Who are "long-term non-progressors"?

A group of individuals with documented HIV infection as early as the late 1970s and early 1980s currently have no evidence of AIDS and have normal CD4 counts. These HIV-infected persons have been called "long-term non-progressors" (or long-term survivors) and detailed studies of their immune systems have been initiated.

While a unified explanation as to why these individuals have not progressed to AIDS has not emerged, several factors characterize this group. First, they have a low virus load. Second, initial evidence suggests that these individuals are more likely to have HIV strains less virulent than strains infecting others. Third, high levels of antibodies that may neutralize HIV are more likely to be found in this group. Fourth, production of chemicals and cells thought to play a role in inhibiting HIV replication may be more active in these persons compared with those individuals progressing to AIDS. A recent finding that the frequency of a certain genetic marker (termed CKR5 deletion) was significantly elevated in those who had survived HIV-1 infection for more than 10 years emphasizes an additional factor that may delay progression to AIDS among certain individuals who are infected with the virus.

121. Do some infections accelerate progression to AIDS?

Infectious agents have also been proposed as cofactors in the development of AIDS. However, there is, at this time, no conclusive evidence that any factor other than HIV is either necessary for or contributes to the acceleration of symptoms of AIDS patients.

122. Do any adult groups differ significantly in their course of HIV infection from others?

The primary determinant of HIV disease progression and survival is HIV viral levels in the body. Other factors unrelated to virus, its therapy, or the treatment of its complications have little direct influence on the course of HIV disease. An important study of patients in a large AIDS clinic found no difference in the rate of disease progression or survival related to sex, race, injection drug use, or socioeconomic status. A key contribution of this study was the access to standardized care across all risk groups. There is little reason to believe that patients who receive similar care will experience differences in disease progression or death as a result of their use of drugs, socieconomic group, sex, or race.

The study also found, as reported by other investigators, that increased age was associated with a more rapid progression of disease and lower survival than in younger patients. The precise reasons for accelerated disease progression in older patients are unclear, although limited evidence suggests that these individuals may have a decreased capacity to produce CD4 lymphocytes when compared with younger individuals.

123. How does the approach of AIDS patients to the terminal stages of their illness affect their treatment decisions?

The rapid evolution of therapy for HIV raises hope that the poor prognosis for these patients will be improved. Nonetheless, at this time no treatment has been shown to prevent death from AIDS even though death is delayed by some available drugs. Many AIDS patients consider their prognosis and weigh it against issues involving the quality of life and discomfort of terminal care. In one survey, 95% of patients wanted hospitalization for pneumonia, a normally treatable condition in AIDS, but only about 55% wanted admission to the Intensive Care Unit and mechanical ventilation if it were required. Only 19% wanted intensive care and mechanical ventilation if they were mentally disabled in the presence of *Pneumocystis carinii* pneumonia and only 17% wanted cardiopulmonary resuscitation in the event of cardiopulmonary arrest.

Many of the patients surveyed had thought about their wishes for terminal care, but only about a third had made their wishes known to their physician. There was no consensus in the survey on when patients preferred these discussions to take place or in which setting. Almost 50% of the patients wanted their partners to make care decisions should the patient become mentally incompetent, 33% wanted family members to make the decision, and only 14% wanted their physician to make the decision. Only 28% of the surveyed patients had prepared a durable power of attorney to designate the person of their choice as the legal decision maker for their care.

Some studies noted a sharply increased suicide rate among AIDS patients. A risk of suicide in excess of 50 times higher than the national average was found in AIDS patients in New York City and California in the mid-1980s. The rate of suicide appears to be declining now, perhaps due to emerging therapies that improve the prognosis for AIDS patients. The suicide rate in AIDS patients decreased to only about seven times that for a comparable population from 1987 to 1989 in the United States.

124. Can children infected with HIV be vaccinated for other infectious diseases as is done with uninfected children?

Children receive vaccinations for a variety of infectious diseases. These vaccines contain live, attenuated, or inactivated microorganisms that evoke an immune response against a pathogen without creating disease. Although the vast majority of children have no difficulty with these treatments, a small number do have adverse reactions after vaccination because of immune suppression. Many physicians are therefore concerned about the risk of introducing live or attenuated microorganisms via vaccination into children who harbor HIV because these children may be more susceptible to adverse effects from the vaccines than uninfected children. The CDC published guidelines in 1987 which were revised in 1988 and still remain current regarding immunization practices in the United States for HIV-infected children.

Vaccination procedures for HIV-infected children are based on the presence or absence of symptoms. The CDC recommends standard vaccination procedures for asymptomatic children with one exception. Because many HIV-infected children come from homes with others infected with HIV, inactivated polio vaccine rather than live virus polio vaccine should be given. There is a risk that either the child or immune suppressed persons in the household without immunity to polio could develop disease from the live virus vaccine.

Symptomatic children should also avoid live polio virus vaccine and other attenuated vaccines, including BCG, a vaccine containing live bacteria sometimes used to prevent tuberculosis. The MMR (mumps-measles-rubella) vaccine is an exception. It contains attenuated virus and has been shown to be safe in these children. Other vaccines containing inactivated organisms, such as DPT (diphtheria, pertussis, tetanus) and Hib (*Haemophilus influenza* b) are safe and should be administered as in children without HIV infection. The CDC also recommends that symptomatic HIV-infected children receive an annual influenza vaccination and all HIV-infected children 2 years of age or older receive a one-time injection of pneumococcal vaccine. After known exposures to chicken pox and measles, the CDC recommends administration of immune globulin to prevent these illnesses which may be devastating in immune compromised people.

125. Is it possible to develop a vaccine against HIV?

There are several difficulties in developing a vaccine against HIV not frequently encountered in the development of vaccines against other viral diseases. The purpose of a vaccine is to create immunity against a microorganism, in this case HIV, before infection occurs. A vaccine can be a virus or a component of a virus altered to lose its disease-producing properties while retaining enough of its unique chemical structure to evoke an immune response in the host. The immune response that results can protect the host from later infection. Vaccines act like the natural infection by stimulating long-lasting immunity to the microorganism. This strategy requires a structure that shares features with all strains of the virus being vaccinated against and to which the immune response can be directed. Successful vaccines generate an immune response aimed at the infectious agent, and this response prepares the immune system to respond to subsequent infection.

HIV presents significant challenges to these requirements for a successful vaccine. An invariant portion of the virus against which an immune response can be directed is an elusive goal. HIV generates different strains quickly, not only between infected individuals, but within the same infected person. Even the production of a family of vaccines that together cover the majority of subtypes is a difficult goal.

In addition to an ill-defined best target, the most desirable immune response against that target is not established. Scientists are working to understand the merits of vaccines that generate solely antibodies versus cell-mediated immunity. Both of these vaccine strategies have advantages and disadvantages that may not be evident in a laboratory setting, and can only be identified through clinical testing.

A candidate vaccine must prove safe and effective. The challenges of conducting large-scale field tests that quickly prove the efficacy of a candidate HIV vaccine are unprecedented in vaccine development. The choice of an appropriate population is the first difficulty. Choosing seronegative members of high-risk groups runs the risk of including infected subjects who are misclassified by testing at the outset of the study. Findings from these subjects would complicate the efficacy claims of the vaccine if their infection became evident during the course of the trial. Subjects willing to participate in a vaccine study may pay great attention to behavioral changes that make them less susceptible to HIV infection. If this is the case, thousands of patients would need to be enrolled and followed for several years before the effects of the vaccine could be established. Choosing a population not at risk for HIV infection requires even more observation before sufficient numbers were exposed to virus allowing evaluation of the effects of the vaccine.

A final requirement for the efficacy testing of a vaccine is defining an adequate response. Surely the prevention of clinical illness is a minimum prerequisite for success, but it is unclear if preventing infection altogether or allowing HIV infection but preventing clinical illness are acceptable endpoints. Only years of observation will show that despite infection, patients benefit from vaccination by preventing or slowing clinically evident disease.

Some progress has been made towards a vaccine. Humans exposed to several candidate vaccines generate an immune response. None of these subjects was then challenged with HIV, and a scientifically sanctioned deliberate challenge will not take place for ethical reasons. Animal models testing SIV vaccines protect against infection in some laboratory conditions, but many years of work lie ahead before scientists will create a vaccine that is both safe and effective in humans.

126. What is the process that leads to new drugs?

The process of developing and licensing new drugs for sale to the public is highly regulated by the federal government. In the United States, the ultimate responsibility to evaluate the effectiveness and safety of new drugs before approving a drug for use rests with the Food and Drug Administration, or FDA. Before a drug is released for research purposes, a sponsoring company, organization or individual must file an Investigational New Drug Application (IND) with the FDA or the appropriate national agency for countries other than the United States. The IND contains detailed information on the plan to investigate the compound in humans along with information from work completed in animals suggesting that administration to humans poses an acceptable risk.

After approval from the FDA to begin studies through an IND, new drugs are first given to volunteers who may or may not be patients in studies that are called Phase I trials. These first studies establish how the drug behaves in the body and the duration of its presence before it is cleared from the bloodstream. These typically very small studies examine the safety of the compound by gradual increases in dose with intense observation after exposure to the compound. Once the drug's initial characteristics are known, it will be studied in larger numbers of patients in Phase II trials, with the goal of demonstrating that the drug has the suspected activity.

After the completion of Phase II trials, large numbers of patients are treated with the compound in Phase III trials. These trials usually include large numbers of patients; they are designed to establish the effectiveness of the compound and to verify that the drug is safe. All of the clinical data and all other relevant information are then gathered into a New Drug Application (NDA). This document is submitted to the FDA or appropriate agency outside of the United States for approval to market the drug.

Determining the safety and efficacy of the compound is often a difficult task. Desperately ill patients with few or no therapeutic options, as is true for many AIDS patients, often opt to accept risks not usually permissible for patients who are less ill or for whom effective therapies exist. No approved AIDS therapy is risk free, and many of the effective licensed compounds have toxicities not normally acceptable in patients who do not have life-threatening illnesses. Efficacy is also sometimes difficult to determine. Drugs that lengthen survival compared with no treatment, or that are at least as effective as other existing treatments, are truly efficacious. Some drugs may not lengthen survival, but may enhance a patient's quality of life or have other benefits that may warrant their use.

In recognition of the paucity of treatments for AIDS patients, pharmaceutical companies and federal regulators have greatly sped the development process, and compressed clinical trial durations and review times from those typically encountered. The FDA established innovative procedures to speed access to promising new drugs by allowing expanded access to investigational drugs under certain circumstances. The FDA has attempted to identify early, but incomplete, laboratory evidence that a drug may be efficacious and then release the drug to physicians on that basis. All approved drugs for the treatment of HIV infection were released to the public much earlier than normal through a variety of accelerated procedures.

127. What experimental approaches to treat HIV infection are under investigation?

A variety of different compounds that may possibly benefit those with AIDS are under investigation. Compounds chemically related to new nucleoside reverse transcriptase inhibitors are in varying stages of development; although these new compounds may be superior to those already in use, there seems little reason to believe that they will represent major advances or successfully avoid all of the toxicities that plague the reverse transcriptase inhibitors already in use.

Physicians are researching another set of molecules called non-nucleoside reverse transcriptase inhibitors. These compounds inhibit reverse transcriptase as do the nucleoside analogues, but the inhibition is different. Early studies proved the drugs to be relatively safe, however the virus readily mutated to develop highly resistant strains after only a few weeks on the drug. The future use of these drugs is uncertain, although they may have a role when used in combination with other compounds.

Another set of compounds called protease inhibitors hold great promise in the therapy of AIDS. Advance-generation protease inhibitors that are more active and more easily administered than the available protease inhibitors are in development. Many other compounds that are not specifically directed against HIV are also under investigation. Immune system-enhancing compounds called cytokines, biological response modifiers including interferon, therapeutic vaccines that stimulate the immune system of already infected persons, and other compounds found fortuitously to inhibit HIV in the laboratory, are under study. At present, none of these latter compounds is thought to be a major therapeutic advance that will radically alter the course of AIDS. There is also much interest in identifying therapies that will prevent opportunistic infections regardless of the existence of effective antiretroviral therapy. At this time, prophylaxis of opportunistic infections is limited to *Pneumocystis carnii* and *Mycobacterium avium* disease. Efforts are underway to develop the best prophylactic regimen active against other opportunistic infections.

128. Where is AIDS research conducted?

Many institutions and groups participate in a diverse array of AIDS research initiatives. Government and private institutions, both for profit and nonprofit, address a number of different aspects of AIDS in many different countries. Government work, especially in the United States, has supported three broad fronts. As is its tradition, the National Institutes of Health (NIH) of the United States supports research at NIH and other institutions to enhance understanding of the basic science of HIV and the immune response to it. This laboratory work does not involve direct care of patients but does serve as a basis for therapeutic advances. The NIH also funds a large effort devoted to the development of a vaccine for HIV.

In a similar fashion, the NIH funds physicians at other institutions to conduct clinical trials. These trials are designed to identify new therapies for HIV infection and the illnesses that accompany it. Much of the government funding for clinical research passes through the Division of AIDS (DAIDS) in the National Institute for Allergy and Infectious Disease. DAIDS coordinates the AIDS Clinical Trial Group (ACTG), a group of United States medical centers where a wide range of AIDS clinical research is conducted.

Some European countries (e.g., The United Kingdom, the Netherlands, and France) have a similar approach to AIDS research. The precise focus of government sponsored research in these countries may vary somewhat from research sponsored by the United States government.

Research completed by private organizations falls into two broad categories, for-profit and not-for-profit. The pharmaceutical and biotechnology industry performs most of the for-profit research on AIDS in the world. This industry devotes millions of dollars to efforts directed at developing new therapies for the treatment of AIDS and its related conditions. The pharmaceutical industry is the principal source of new drugs and the primary manufacturer of presently licensed compounds. Its efforts range from basic science to clinical trials, and much of this work is done in conjunction with academic researchers.

Not-for-profit organizations usually funnel donations to research efforts that address their particular interest. Some sponsor laboratory work, some clinical work, and others support medical education and policy research. Some well-recognized groups include The American Foundation for AIDS Research, Project Inform, The Arthur Ashe Foundation, The Gay Men's Health Crisis, The Physicians Association for AIDS Care, The Magic Johnson Foundation, and the Pediatric AIDS Foundation. Many nonprofit organizations involved in HIV and AIDS activities accept donations offered in support of their interests.

129. How does the United States government fund HIV research?

In 1982, the first year funds were formally budgeted for AIDS, $8 million was designated for AIDS. Until 1986, much of the funding for AIDS was redirected from other research projects within the budget of the NIH and the CDC. In 1996, Congress budgeted $7.27 billion to combat AIDS through a variety of programs and planned substantial increases for 1997.

AIDS funding in 1996 gave $2.87 billion to the Public Health Service which distributed $1.4 billion in grants to academic centers and other agencies, in large part, through the NIH. About $584 million was targeted for prevention programs consisting primarily of risk reduction and educational programs conducted by state and local organizations; $762 million was spent for treatment programs. As part of the public health service appropriation, the FDA received about $72 million for research.

Besides the monies appropriated for the public health service, additional federal agencies receive funding for AIDS-related services and activities. Medicaid, a federal program that funds medical care for some low-income individuals, received $1.5 billion for treatment payments. Medicare, a federal program for the elderly, received $690 million for AIDS health care. Other federal programs including Social Security, the Veterans Administration, The Bureau of Prisons, and the Defense Department also received money for the prevention and treatment of HIV-related disease.

The $2.87 billion provided to the Public Health Service for AIDS-related activities compares with $2.11 billion for cancer research, treatment and prevention, $829 million for heart disease research, treatment, and prevention, and $325 million for the same activities related to diabetes.

130. How does one learn about clinical studies with new drugs and therapies?

A clinical trial assesses the safety and efficacy of a drug or therapy for the treatment of a specific clinical condition. Often conducted at large medical centers and involving collaboration of many physicians and patients, these trials are sometimes also performed by a patient's primary physician depending on the condition under study.

Clinical trials that may lead to new claims for either new or existing drugs or therapies are conducted under the aegis of a national health authority. In the United States, this authority is the FDA which codifies the standards and ethics for clinical research in the United States. Other countries have similar arrangements that may differ in practice, but still fulfill the same role as the FDA.

The following sources list information on clinical trials and new AIDS treatments:

- AIDS Clinical Trials Information Services (ACTIS) provides information of experimental clinical trials with drugs to treat HIV. This service is reached at (800) TRIALS-A [(800) 874-2572].

- AIDS Treatment Data Network is located at 611 Broadway, Suite 613, New York, NY 10012, (212) 260-8868 or (800) 734-7104.

- The *American Foundation for AIDS Research (AMFAR) AIDS/HIV Treatment Directory* contains current HIV/AIDS treatment information, clinical drug research protocols available nationwide, compassionate use and expanded access programs, state drug assistance program information, pharmaceutical drug assistance and other available printed information. Contact AMFAR at 733 Third Ave., 12th Floor, New York, NY 10017-3204, (212) 682-7440; subscription line (800) 38-AMFAR; (212) 682-9812 Fax.

- The National Library of Medicine (NLM) offers online computer information on medical topics (MEDLINE) and AIDS-related (AIDSLINE) topics. Information on access is available at http://www.nlm.nih.gov or (800) 638-8480.

- Project Inform's Treatment Information is located at 1965 Market St., Suite 220, San Francisco, CA 94103, (415) 558-8669, (800) 822-7422 (hotline), (415) 558-0684 Fax. It offers access to current treatment information for HIV disease.

131. How can one evaluate alternative treatments for HIV infection?

Alternative treatments are therapies that are not usually used in traditional medicine. Many individuals with HIV infection use alternative therapies to supplement or replace licensed drugs. Often family, friends, or patient advocacy organizations tell AIDS patients about untraditional treatments that may offer hope but are difficult to evaluate because of limited information on their use or medical effects. The following guidelines can assist in discriminating therapies that may have some utility in the treatment of HIV infection from those that are either fraudulent or that have no reasonable basis to be active against HIV:

1. Studies evaluating the activity of the compound should be published in peer-reviewed journals that maintain high scientific standards. It is not true that scientifically valid studies of alternative therapies will not be published in these journals. Patients should never accept a promoter's statement that studies have been published; copies of those studies should be requested.

    Some groups allege that the medical establishment attempts to suppress good therapies to profit from the treatments that are already in use. Any effective therapy for any disease that causes suffering would be welcomed by practitioners of traditional medicine. Many medicines that are today viewed as traditional were discovered by screening natural products or by adopting practices by indigenous peoples who do not practice Western medicine.

2. Anecdotal reports of successful clinical outcomes should always be treated with skepticism. Personal testimonies are often used by promoters of products in the absence of detailed information demonstrating the scientific testing of the compound. Reports that individuals feel better while receiving a therapy does not prove that the therapy is effective. The strong desire to feel better may help a person to believe that the medication is working even though there is no objective evidence that the compound has contributed any measurable clinical improvement. Anecdotal information should always be supplemented with other information that suggests that the compound may work. The most valid indicators of the activity of a prospective compound are evidence of a change in laboratory tests, a decreased frequency of opportunistic infection, and prolonged survival of patients who have received the drug under circumstances in which the survival can be assessed properly.

3. Other sources should be consulted before making a decision to use a new, unproved therapy. Organizations or individuals who have no financial interest in the product or treatment may help to assess its potential benefit; the promoter of the compound may not have a similarly disinterested view of the drug.

4. One should always understand what the treatment actually is. Any promoter of a product claiming secret ingredients should be treated with great skepticism. There is no reason why compounds must be held secretly because patents that protect the owner of the drug are readily obtained.

5. One should always attempt to understand the price of the treatment. If compounds are expensive because a major investment was required to discover and develop the product, then the high price may be warranted. Untested, untraditional drugs or treatments do not require the same costs for their development and therefore should cost less than traditional drugs or treatments.

6. Any treatment promoted as a cure must be thoroughly investigated. Rigorously documented evidence that the therapy is indeed curative should be demanded.

7. Travel to a foreign country to receive a new treatment should raise several questions in the mind of a prospective patient. The claim that a particular clinic in another country has discovered a major treatment for HIV infection should prompt questions why the new treatment has not been imported, presented at international meetings on HIV infection, or published in the scientific literature.

8. The promoter of any new treatment should always be interviewed. The prospective patient should always establish the qualifications of this person to evaluate the new drug.

9.   Therapies that are claimed to treat many different illnesses simultaneously are often fraudulent.

10. If other drugs that the patient is receiving must be stopped to begin the new treatment, the patient and his or her physician should determine why this is necessary.

CHAPTER EIGHT

HIV and Public Policy

132. How did HIV and AIDS initially impact public policy?

When public policy first started forming in response to the spread of HIV in the early 1980s, legislators and health care professionals were uncertain as to what policies were appropriate for HIV infection and AIDS. Traditionally, the public health model used in the battle against the spread of a transmissible disease, particularly a sexually transmitted disease, is to identify and cure the affected person. During the first few years of the AIDS epidemic, when the transmissible nature of the disease was known, there was no test for the infectious agent and thus, no way to determine who appeared healthy yet was infected. In addition, following development of antibody testing to identify infected individuals, no treatments could be offered until ZDV (zidovudine) became available in 1987. Although ZDV was useful in the treatment of HIV infection in selected individuals, it was not curative. Further, because of the social taboos against some of the primary modes of transmission (e.g., use of injecting drugs and homosexual sex), and because of fears of infection through casual contact, those individuals with HIV infection or AIDS were further stigmatized. HIV infection and AIDS had important implications for the potential of infected people to lose jobs and health insurance, as well as to endanger relationships among friends and family.

The uniqueness of HIV infection and AIDS as a medical condition and the powerful social issues that surrounded infected individuals set HIV/AIDS apart from any other disease. Recognizing the need to develop public policies to deal with the needs of society and the infected individual, makers of public policy formed a doctrine known as "HIV Exceptionalism." This doctrine acknowledged that the traditional medical model used in transmissible diseases could not apply to HIV/AIDS and that public policies be designed to reflect this fact. The absence of a cure, the recognition that infected but overtly healthy individuals could infect others, the ability to identify infected individuals through antibody testing, and the significant social issues surrounding the disease meant that public policies needed to be designed, in part, to address some of the unique issues raised by the HIV/AIDS epidemic.

133. Can results of an HIV antibody test be given to public officials?

In the early years of the HIV/AIDS epidemic, many states created publicly funded sites that offered confidential or anonymous HIV-antibody testing to provide an environment that was perceived as safe for those seeking testing. With anonymous testing, the identity of the person being tested is unknown and the results are often relayed to the person tested by a numbered coding system. With confidential testing, the identity of the person tested is known to the health care provider or designee but kept a secret from others. The practice of offering anonymous and confidential testing was a major influence in encouraging those who might be intimidated by the social stigma surrounding HIV infection to be tested. Within the last few years, a growing number of states have passed legislation requiring testing centers to divulge to state health officials the name of any person who tests HIV-antibody positive. Proponents of this practice believe that such reporting facilitates prevention efforts and allows for the tracing and potential contacting of sexual partners of infected individuals (termed "contact tracing"). Others believe that mandatory reporting of names to state health officials could prevent a person who might otherwise be tested from seeking testing and receiving appropriate medical attention and education.

Both discrimination of those who are HIV infected and episodes of unlawful breaches of confidential HIV test results are additional concerns involved in the mandatory reporting of names to public health officials.

Before seeking HIV-antibody testing, an individual should obtain a special understanding of whether their testing is anonymous and/or confidential. If anonymous testing is required by the person tested, one could conceivably travel to a state that permits anonymous testing, or purchase a home collection antibody test kit. Home collection test kits, approved by the FDA in 1996, are purchased in a pharmacy and require the deposit of a sample of blood through a pin prick onto a collection card. This card, with a unique bar code that identifies the individual test kit but not the person tested, is then mailed to the testing center. Results are obtained by telephone and, if positive, telephone counseling and referral are provided by the testing center.

134. Under what circumstances can sexual or other high-risk contacts of persons with HIV be notified by public officials?

Contact tracing, also called partner notification, is the process by which public health agencies identify sexual or other high-risk contacts of a person with a sexually transmitted disease. Originally used for syphilis and gonorrhea, states now extend this process to HIV infection. Some states ask that the infected individual notify his or her contacts, other states ask that the names of partners by volunteered for referral to trained public health workers. The identity of the referring, infected person is not disclosed to the sexual contact who is notified.

In 1988, 12 states had policies requiring the notification of known partners of HIV-infected people. By 1996, all states were required to have a partner notification system as a requirement to receive federal funding to support HIV counseling and testing at publicly funded sites. Colorado, Idaho, and North Carolina ask public health workers to identify, trace, notify, and counsel volunteered partners. California, Florida, Georgia, Hawaii, Illinois, South Carolina, and Washington follow the same procedures but only for contacts who fall into designated risk groups. Maryland and Oregon require health professionals to notify contacts if the patient does not do this voluntarily. Other states, including California, Florida, Georgia, Illinois, Indiana, Maryland, Michigan, Mississippi, North Dakota, Pennsylvania, Rhode Island, Tennessee, and Wisconsin require notification of funeral personnel and emergency room staff exposed during work to infected patients. Most of these programs rely on the accurate volunteering of information by an infected person, but many with HIV infection may not divulge the names of their contacts for a number of reasons.

A study compared the success of different forms of notification with patients who provided names of both sexual and drug partners. Trained counselors successfully contacted 50% of partners compared with successful contacts in only 7% of cases when the patient himself attempted to notify a partner. Of all notified contacts, 50% were tested for HIV and 25% of these people were found to be infected. Decisions to use public health versus patient notification requires an analysis of cost, confidentiality, possible discrimination, and the "duty to warn."

The duty to warn someone at significant risk for HIV infection who has otherwise not been informed is the one clear circumstance in which there is legal precedent to breech the confidentiality of an infected person. In many states, confidentiality laws involving HIV status have been amended to allow physicians or other health care workers to inform an identified third party that they had been exposed by an unnamed party. Many statutes also allow a physician to pass such information on to local health authorities who then contact the third party to impart the information that he or she may have had a critical exposure to HIV. Physicians and other health care workers who know of a person's HIV status are otherwise obligated to respect the confidentiality of this information. It is less clear if a health care worker can disclose information to another health care worker about a patient's HIV infection status. Many, but not all, jurisdictions allow medical personnel to divulge the HIV status of a patient to another health care worker if such knowledge is important to the care of the patient.

135. Can life insurance companies require an individual to obtain HIV-antibody testing as a condition for granting insurance?

The legality of requiring that an individual take an HIV-antibody test as a pre-condition for purchase of insurance depends upon where a person lives and on the type of insurance purchased. When health, life, or disability insurance is obtained as part of a group policy, such as commonly occurs in an employment situation, it is unlikely that information on HIV status would be requested. However, more latitude is given to insurance companies who request such information to sell insurance to persons through individual policies. In this setting, and particularly with life insurance, there is an increased likelihood that HIV status information will be requested as a condition to purchase the policy. In nearly all cases, HIV infection precludes individuals from acquiring life insurance.

If an HIV-infected person seeks health insurance after their status is known, there are several ways to acquire such coverage. One method to obtain health insurance is through a group plan in an employment setting, or by purchasing an individual policy if residing in a state that offers "high-risk pool insurance." Such insurance allows for a set number of "slots" available to people who are diagnosed with a life-threatening illness but who have been turned down as "uninsurable" by private companies. Not all states have high-risk pool insurance and information about availability and procedures to apply can usually be obtained from a local hospital social worker or HIV/AIDS organization.

136. Can HIV-antibody testing be used to deny employment?

Before federal legislation enacted in 1990, many states had laws that prohibited an otherwise qualified person with a disability or handicap from having that information used to determine eligibility for or continuation of employment. In most cases, HIV/AIDS was included in the definition of a disability or handicap and these laws precluded employers from requesting or using HIV status to determine eligibility for employment.

In 1990, the Americans with Disabilities Act was signed into law. This federal law prohibits employment discrimination against otherwise qualified persons with a disability. All stages of HIV infection, including asymptomatic illness, are included within the definition of a disability. An exception to federal protection of HIV-infected persons from discrimination in employment situations is the requirement of mandatory testing and exclusion of infected persons from employment in the United States military, Peace Corps, and Foreign Service.

While the Americans with Disabilities Act has been used successfully to provide protection and redress against discrimination in employment settings, it has also played an important role in allowing HIV-infected persons proper access to medical treatment. While fortunately an uncommon occurrence, some medical and dental facilities have refused to treat persons based on HIV status and these facilities have been successfully sued under protections offered by the Americans with Disabilities Act.

137. Can people be discharged from the United States military because of their HIV status?

Although HIV infection precludes entrance into the military, existing military personnel who are infected are not discharged but are placed in a non-combat role. The changing nature of how the federal government perceives the role of military personnel with HIV infection is reflected by a provision that was passed by Congress in 1996. This provision allowed HIV-infected people to be discharged from the military based on the theory that they would not be as combat-ready as other troops. This provision was then repealed a short time later by Congress. As with many areas of HIV policy, this matter is not completely settled and is subject to sensitive shifts in the political atmosphere.

138. What role does quarantine play in reducing the spread of HIV?

Quarantining imposes restrictions, sometimes geographic, on a person to prevent transmission of an infectious disease. The American College of Physicians and the Infectious Diseases Society of America issued a joint position paper early in the AIDS crisis analyzing quarantining as a means to address the AIDS epidemic. These groups concluded that the systematic quarantining of HIV-infected people was impractical and unsound both medically and ethically. Their reasoning was strongly supported by several observations.

Quarantining is an unjustified invasion of individual liberty and privacy with no medical benefit to society. The practice of quarantining would most likely cause many physicians to not report AIDS cases to health officials to avoid isolation measures for their patients. Failure to report these AIDS cases would alter collection of data important to track the epidemic and to improve understanding of the diseases.

Asymptomatic persons probably account for more cases of HIV transmission than those who are symptomatic. Aside from ethical issues, quarantining only patients with AIDS would not accomplish the desired end of segregating infected people since the majority of those able to transmit HIV infection are without symptoms and are not easily identified. Quarantining all infected patients would require the confinement of over one million Americans. In addition, quarantining persons with AIDS or HIV infection would convey a false sense of security to some who might believe that the risk of becoming infected was reduced and therefore take fewer precautions to avoid infection. They also note that confining individuals who engage in behaviors that transmit HIV will not control a larger epidemic. Last, the logistics of testing, the possibility of inaccurate test results, and the housing of all infected patients makes widespread quarantining impractical and impossible to complete.

139. Are there laws against intentionally transmitting HIV?

There has been a growing trend to criminalize the intentional transmission of HIV from one person to another, particularly by sexual means. Some proposals also have been drafted to include punishment for HIV-infected persons who engage in sexual relations without first divulging their HIV status to their sexual partner (such a statute was proposed in California in 1996). While such statutes may appear gratifying at first glance, they are not easily applied from a legal perspective. To prosecute such cases would require specific proof that involvement with the accused was the only possible way by which a victim could have become infected. Further, making it a crime for an HIV-infected person to have sex with an uninfected person without divulging one's HIV status presents a different challenge of acquiring adequate legal evidence.

140. What are guidelines for HIV-infected children in school?

There is no known case of a child acquiring HIV infection through casual contact at school, day care, or foster care settings. While school attendance of HIV-infected children has been a source of controversy in the United States, most courts have upheld the right of these children to attend school and forbid discrimination directed against them. The United States Public

Health Service issued the following recommendations in 1985 defining policies for education of these children, and these guidelines remain applicable today:

- Behavior, neurological development, physical condition, and the expected interaction with other children should dictate the educational procedures and care of infected children. A team including the child's physician, public health personnel, the child's parent, and any personnel teaching or delivering care for the child can best decide appropriate educational circumstances for the student after weighing risks and benefits in the proposed setting.

- The benefits of an unrestricted school setting outweigh disadvantages for most school-age infected children. Disadvantages include theoretical but not previously observed transmission of HIV to other children, but more probable is the transmission of childhood infections from healthy children to a child with AIDS.

- A restricted environment may be appropriate for infected preschoolers and some children with neurological handicaps who are unable to control body secretions or who bite. Children with open, oozing lesions may also require a restricted environment.

- Only persons aware of the child's infection should deliver care that may place them in contact with body fluids and excrement as encountered during changing diapers and feeding. Other safety precautions include following good hand-washing practices after exposure to body fluids and using gloves when the caretaker has open skin lesions. Any open lesions on the child should also be covered.

- All schools, regardless of the attendance of children with HIV, should adopt procedures for handling blood and body fluids. Soiled surfaces should be cleansed promptly with disinfectant. Household bleach diluted at one part bleach to ten parts water is a suitable disinfectant.

- Disposable towels or tissues should be used whenever possible, and mops should be rinsed in disinfectant.

- Regular evaluations of the child's hygienic practices should be required. Some children will improve their practices as they mature, but some children will have increasing difficulty maintaining appropriate standards as their health deteriorates.

- Mandatory screening for HIV-antibody testing before school entry is not warranted based on accumulated data.

- Persons caring for infected children must respect the child's privacy, including the maintenance of confidential health records. Only individuals who must know the child's condition should be informed.

- All educational and public health departments are urged to supply parents, children, and educators accurate information to maintain a good educational environment while minimizing the risk of illness to all.

These recommendations were offered by the Public Health Service to guide parents and educators in structuring a safe educational environment. The National Association of State Boards of Education (NASBE) has published a guide for educators to develop effective policies for HIV-infected staff and students. This guide is endorsed by the Centers for Disease Control and Prevention. Entitled, *Someone at School Has AIDS: Guide to Developing Policies for Students and School Staff*

Members Who Are Infected with HIV, it is available from ANSBE, Publications Department, 1012 Cameron Street, Alexandria, VA 22314, telephone (703) 684-4000.

141. What educational efforts are being made in public schools to decrease risk of HIV infection among adolescents?

A large number of adolescents engage in risk behaviors for HIV and AIDS. A recent report evaluated risk factors over a reporting period in 1994 and estimated that nationwide, 2.2% of United States students in grades 9-12 had injected steroids without a doctor's prescription, 1.4% had injected illegal drugs, and more than half had sexual intercourse. The percentage of students who had sexual intercourse with four or more partners was 18.8%. Among those students who were currently sexually active (sexual intercourse during the three months preceding the study), 52% reported that they or their partner had used a condom and 18% reported that they or their partner used birth control pills.

Because adolescents are enrolled in school, educational programs in this setting have been considered potential interventions that can decrease the risk of HIV transmission to and by this group. In 1994, the United States Public Health Service noted that HIV-prevention programs were required in 78% of states and 83% of school districts; such programs were required in 85% of all middle/junior and senior high schools. Although no official figures are currently available, anecdotal information suggests that over 90% of United States school districts currently require HIV-prevention education for students. All states that require HIV-prevention education currently provide in-service training for teachers on this subject. Of school districts that require HIV-prevention education, around 60% provide such training.

142. Where is information available on legal issues and AIDS?

The Lambda Legal Defense and Educational Fund-AIDS Clearinghouse, 666 Broadway, New York, NY 10012, telephone (212) 995-8585 is a national organization that maintains a national clearinghouse for AIDS and the law, including legislation and materials relevant to litigation. Lambda publishes *AIDS Update*, a monthly review of AIDS-related legal materials. *AIDS Policy and Law*, available from LRP Publications, (800) 341-7874, is a biweekly newsletter that focuses on current policy and litigation surrounding AIDS. In many cases, technical questions are best left to an appropriately trained professional who can interpret the law and discuss specific issues.

143. What is the economic impact of AIDS in the United States?

AIDS imposes huge costs on society. Medical care, AIDS education, research to understand and develop treatments for AIDS, and blood screening are all direct costs attributable to AIDS. More subtle costs include earnings that are lost by mostly young patients and the productivity that goes with it, disruption to families, funding directed away from other illnesses, and the emotional toll paid by millions as their friends and loved ones suffer.

The prolonged and multifaceted nature of AIDS makes it one of the most expensive of all diseases. Estimates of the first 10,000 American AIDS patients are telling. These patients averaged 166 days in the hospital for medical costs of $140,000 per patient. An average of $19,000 of income was lost during the 360 days these patients remained away from work on account of AIDS, and future earnings lost averaged $460,000 per patient. The overall economic impact of these 10,000 patients, excluding research funding and educational costs, was about $6.3 billion from direct medical expenses.

Improvements in the treatment of AIDS and less lengthy hospital stays reduced the direct cost in 1996 to about $40,000 per patient per year, totaling approximately $110,000 over the life of a patient. The direct medical costs of new cases and previously diagnosed cases in 1997 are estimated to total in excess of $6 billion, not including lost employment, reduced productivity, shortened life expectancy, social services, research, and antibody testing of blood donations. The total also does not include the care of HIV-infected patients without AIDS. In addition, the advent of protease inhibitor therapy that may increase survival of those with AIDS means that current projections of the lifetime cost of treating patients with AIDS are underestimations.

Treating AIDS is more expensive than treating most other illnesses. A disproportionate share of AIDS care is funded by government programs and not by private insurance; in many cases, AIDS care remains unpaid. The shift to increased public financing is a grave concern. Studies document that low reimbursement by Medicaid increases expenses to Medicaid encouraging reliance on better reimbursed hospital care and not on less expensive outpatient care. The growing expense of treating AIDS poses great economic challenges when health care cost containment is more important than ever.

Moving care away from hospitals to less expensive settings that can meet the needs of the patient is an important means in reducing the cost of care. An early study determined that 15% of 273 surveyed patients could leave the hospital at least once in the terminal stages of disease if a spouse, friend, or family member could accommodate their needs. The absence of a suitable caretaker at home eliminates home care as an option for many patients. An example that is becoming more typical with time is the plight of AIDS babies. A survey taken between 1981 and 1986, and relevant today, found that many lacked homes because of abandonment or because the mother herself was homeless, disabled, or dead. These children remained in the hospital four times longer than those with homes, independent of their medical condition. Community health services may improve these situations and reduce costs, but communities vary in the amount of planning and degree of implementation of those plans. Finally, there are many patients who may not be appropriate for this form of care; they will continue to challenge the health care delivery system and shrinking budgets.

Besides the direct costs of treating those with AIDS that result from treatment, research, and education, there are other less tangible costs associated with this epidemic. Because HIV infection and AIDS have impacted people who are young, the years of productive life lost is greater with AIDS than with other diseases more common among the elderly. This means that society loses not only the years of tax-paying revenue from these people but, more importantly, the productivity of their creativity and the contributions they may have made to society. In this respect, there is simply no true measurement of the economic loss suffered by society from an epidemic such as this.

144. What are some of the ethical and social issues posed by the AIDS epidemic?

AIDS and HIV infection pose immense problems not only for people affected directly by the disease, but also for society at large. Because the illness is transmissible, much debate over appropriate methods to prevent spread of the virus has taken place. In many respects, careful considerations of facts has taken precedence over drastic action that is unlikely to serve any useful purpose. For example, proposals in the early years of the epidemic for large scale-quarantining of those with AIDS has become irrelevant as the scientific, legal, and ethical issues have become clear. However, the continued spread of HIV has raised additional issues such as the role of mandatory HIV screening for various groups at risk for HIV infection.

Should health care workers be tested and, if so, should their test results be made known to patients? Should patients undergo HIV-antibody testing before a health care worker performs an invasive procedure? Should a pregnant woman be required to take an HIV-antibody test, and if positive, what guarantee to access to treatment for her and her baby should be made? Should minors be permitted to purchase home-collection HIV kits without divulging the test results to their parents? Should a person's HIV status be revealed at the time of their death? Are needle exchange programs effective and how should laws reflect this? With government sponsored programs that provide for a limited number of individuals to have access to drugs, who should get preference?

Because HIV infection is a chronic condition, those with HIV infection will live in the presence of uninfected persons for years. The risk of unwarranted stigmatization and discrimination of those with AIDS by denying access to care, housing, employment, and appropriate social interaction can be reduced by adequate education for all. This education can also serve to better those who develop and implement public policy. Those infected with the virus must also be educated to learn how to prevent spread of HIV; others who are uninfected must learn the same lessons. Procedures followed at the individual level by all people can reduce the social disruption of HIV and minimize the numbers of new infections. The proper teaching of facts of AIDS and disseminating information on how to prevent infection is a constant social issue and one that may have a variety of approaches.

AIDS adds immense financial burdens to an already failing health care delivery system. Not only is care delivered for AIDS expensive, but the redirection of research dollars away from other illnesses carries another cost: the lost opportunities to understand better other illnesses that have not receded in the face of AIDS. Other financial issues that will continue to evolve are the cost and access to insurance for HIV-infected people. It is difficult to imagine a time when the breadth and depth of the ethical and social aspects of HIV and AIDS will not be at least as challenging as it is today.

PERSPECTIVES

There are many poorly understood illnesses in medicine that create immense human suffering. Although AIDS is another entry to this long list, the study of AIDS may ultimately clarify aspects of illnesses as diverse as rheumatoid arthritis, multiple sclerosis, and systemic lupus erythematosus. Each of these diseases and many like them are linked by a common thread, a disorder of immunity. Understanding the immune system better through research related to AIDS may lead to new insights in how these diseases arise and how to treat or prevent them. For the immediate future, however, AIDS will only bring loss.

AIDS was first recognized in 1981 and the virus that causes it in 1983. At that time, patients lived for less than a year after the appearance of an AIDS-defining illness. While many benefit from antiretroviral therapy, the prognosis for those with AIDS is ultimately the same. Most infected with HIV will develop AIDS and all these people will die from AIDS if no other fatal event supervenes. Despite optimism that scientific advances will continue to occur, there is no treatment at present that has been shown to cure HIV infection.

HIV infection is of pandemic proportions. The initial appearance of the virus in well-defined risk groups, such as homosexual men and intravenous drug users in the United States, may have given the impression that HIV infection was limited to people in these groups, but that is not the case. AIDS now appears on all inhabited continents and in people from all walks of life. Just as HIV ignores all geographic boundaries, it also permeates any population that it enters when no precautions are taken to prevent its spread. As of 1996, about 1.5 million Americans were infected, a similar number of Europeans are infected, and in some portions of central Africa up to one-quarter of all people carry HIV. It is possible that large areas of Africa may well be significantly depopulated in the upcoming years as a result of HIV. Not since the 1600s when parts of Europe were devastates by the Black Plague has the world faced a medical challenge of similar proportions.

Even though scientists continue to investigate new drugs and physicians test them in humans, there is no room for complacence. Major therapeutic advances that improve on those currently available may come only in the very indefinite future. Until the existence of a vaccine that has been tested rigorously and proven effective, everyone must consider the possibility of becoming infected with HIV. All must understand how the virus is and is not transmitted, and all must learn the deadly consequences of infection with HIV. All must learn that infection is a lifelong condition that can lead to death and that transmission of that infection exposes their loved ones to a similar fate.

In the absence of effective therapy, education is the only viable option to prevent further cases of HIV infection. AIDS is preventable in nearly every case. Stopping the epidemic is a social concern of course, but in the final analysis, society is composed of individuals. Each person must individually behave in a manner that will halt the spread of the virus. If not one more person were infected, AIDS would become extinct in this generation.

GLOSSARY

ACTG: AIDS Clinical Trials Group, a United States-sponsored federal consortium of academically affiliated clinicians responsible for conducting a large portion of clinical research of AIDS in the United States.

acute: Having a rapid onset, a short course, and pronounced symptoms.

AIDS (Acquired Immunodeficiency Syndrome): The clinical state resulting from prolonged infection with human immunodeficiency virus. It is usually characterized by poorly treatable opportunistic infections and malignancies appearing in the setting of profoundly decreased immunity.

AIDS-related complex (ARC): A syndrome resulting from HIV infection but lacking an opportunistic infection or Kaposi's sarcoma required to meet the case definition of AIDS. Persons with ARC often have chronic systemic symptoms including enlarged lymph nodes, fever, diarrhea, and lethargy along with localized infections. Most people with ARC progress to AIDS; the term ARC, useful at the outset of the epidemic, is now used only infrequently.

AIDS-associated retrovirus (ARV): An early name for HIV no longer in use.

alternative treatment: Therapy with agents that are not approved by a governmental agency.

anemia: A condition marked by a low number of red blood cells and often associated with weakness and fatigue.

ano-genital wart: Raised skin in the anal or genital region occurring as a response to infection with papilloma virus.

antibiotic: A drug that kills or inhibits the growth of microorganisms.

antibody: A protein formed by lymphocytes that reacts against molecules called antigens.

antibody positivity: Possessing antibodies directed against HIV detected by any of several diagnostic tests, although usually by ELISA and confirmed by Western blot testing; synonymous with HIV infection.

antigen: Any substance to which the body responds by producing an immune response.

antiretroviral: A drug active against retroviruses, usually HIV. Antiretrovirals used in humans include zidovudine (ZDV), ddI, ddC, 3TC, d4T, saquinavir, indinavir, nelfinavir, and nevirapine.

aphthous ulcer: Small and painful sores, usually white, that appear inside the mouth.

apoptosis: A process through which cells die in response to a molecular signal; also known as programmed cell death.

arthritis: A clinical condition characterized by inflammation of the joints; it is associated with a large number of different disease processes.

artificial insemination: The introduction of semen into the vagina or uterus to induce pregnancy by nonsexual means.

asymptomatic: Without any subjective evidence of disease or illness.

autologous transfusion: Blood transfusion in which the patient receives his or her own blood, usually donated several weeks before an elective surgical procedure.

AZT: Azidothymidine; also called zidovudine (ZDV). This is an antiretroviral drug that suppresses the replication of HIV.

B lymphocyte: A type of cell involved in normal immunity; B cells produce antibodies.

bacteria: Single-cell organisms that can cause illness when they grow in any part of the body. They are treated with antibiotics.

bDNA: Branched DNA; a laboratory test that uses chemically modified DNA to measure the quantity of HIV RNA (and thus, the number of viral particles) present in body fluids.

benign: Noncancerous, mild.

bisexual: Sexual attraction to both males and females.

blood count: The number of red and white blood cells in the bloodstream.

Candida albicans: A fungus found on the body, in the mouth, and on the genital tracts. Excessive growth of the organism can be associated with clinical symptoms.

candidiasis: A condition produced by infection with *Candida albicans* that can affect the skin, mucous membranes, nails, lungs, gastrointestinal tract, and other tissues.

cardiopulmonary resuscitation: A prescribed sequence of steps to reestablish the breathing and heartbeat in a person in which these have stopped.

carrier: An infected person who shows no signs or symptoms of disease but who harbors a contagious organism.

Centers for Disease Control and Prevention (CDC): A federal agency located in Atlanta, Georgia that plans, conducts, coordinates, and evaluates national programs for the prevention and control of transmissible diseases and other preventable conditions.

CD4 cell: A type of lymphocyte crucial to the normal function of the immune system. Also known as T4 cells, CD4+ lymphocytes and T-helper lymphocytes; they are the principal target cell for HIV infection.

cerebrospinal fluid: The fluid found within the cavities of the brain and surrounding both the brain and the spinal cord.

chemotherapy: A treatment of disease by any drug, although used colloquially most often to refer to the treatment of cancer.

clinical trial: See drug trial.

clotting factors: Proteins essential to blood coagulation found in the bloodstream; absence of these proteins leads to prolonged, sometimes pathological bleeding as in hemophilia.

coccidioidomycosis: An uncommon fungal infection that occurs most frequently in the American Southwest.

colonization: The presence of a microorganism in or on a host without associated disease.

compromised: Lessened, as in an individual's decreased ability to resist infection in compromised immunity.

cross-reactivity: A reaction between an antibody and an antigen that is closely related to, but distinct from, the relevant antigen.

cryoprecipitate: A substance obtained from blood and rich in the clotting factors absent in a common form of hemophilia.

Cryptosporidium: A family of protozoans that causes severe inflammation and diarrhea in AIDS patients.

Cryptococcus neoformans: A fungus that affects the skin, lungs, bones or, most commonly, the nervous system where it causes meningitis.

cytomegalovirus: A virus that is a member of the Herpes family, it causes severe eye infections and gastrointestinal disease in the late stages of AIDS.

dementia: A progressive impairment of intellectual function with marked compromise in at least three of the following areas of mental function: language, memory, visuospatial skills, personality, and cognition.

disorientation: The loss of normal relationship to one's surroundings; particularly the ability to comprehend time, place, and people.

DNA: Deoxyribonucleic acid, a chemical containing genetic information in all living organisms; some viruses also contain DNA as their genetic material.

drug trial: Also known as a clinical trial, the clinical experiment through which researchers determine the effectiveness of different forms of treatment.

ELISA: Enzyme-linked immunosorbent assay, a test employed to detect the presence of HIV antibody.

empirical: Based on observation.

encephalitis: Inflammation of the brain usually due to an infection.

endoscopy: Examination of the inside of the body, usually the intestines or throat, by the use of an instrument called an endoscope.

Epstein-Barr virus: The virus that causes infectious mononucleosis and perhaps other illness in immuno-compromised patients.

esophagitis: Inflammation of the esophagus, the structure that carries food from the mouth to the stomach.

factor VIII: A protein essential for normal blood coagulation; it is deficient in patients with hemophilia type A.

Factor IX: A protein essential for normal blood coagulation; it is deficient in patients with hemophilia type B.

fungi: One-celled organisms in the plant kingdom; some fungi cause disease in persons with altered immunity.

gamma interferon: A protein formed by human cells that limits the production of some viruses.

gastroenteritis: Inflammation or infection of the lining of the stomach or intestines.

gene: The smallest single unit of heritable genetic information; composed of either the nucleic acid DNA or RNA (in some viruses).

gonorrhea: A sexually transmitted disease causing inflammation most often in the genitourinary tract.

helper T lymphocyte: A lymphocyte that bears the CD4 molecule on its surface and is the primary target or HIV infection; also called CD4 lymphocyte.

hematocrit: The volume of red blood cells expressed as a percentage of the total volume of blood.

hemoglobin: A molecule in red blood cells that carries oxygen to cells and carbon dioxide away from cells.

hepatitis B: A virus that causes inflammation of the liver, transmitted through contaminated blood products and sexual exposures.

herpes simplex virus: A virus that usually causes genital and oral lesions; it persists indefinitely in the body after initial infection and reactivates unpredictably.

herpes zoster: Painful, vesicular eruptions on the skin and mucous membranes caused by the varicella zoster virus.

heterosexual: Sexual attraction to the opposite sex.

histoplasmosis: A fungal infection caused by *Histoplasma capsulatum* characterized by fever, swollen glands, cough, weight loss, and anemia. This disease occurs most frequently in the American Midwest.

HIV: Human immunodeficiency virus, the causative agent of AIDS.

HIV antibody positivity: Containing antibodies in the blood directed against HIV; presence of these antibodies are synonymous with HIV infection.

homosexual: Sexual attraction to individuals of one's own sex.

host: An organism on which another organism lives and from which the second organism derives nourishment.

human papillomavirus (HPV): A virus with many different subtypes that causes warts on the skin and venereal warts; the virus has been linked to cervical carcinoma.

HTLV-III: Human T-lymphotropic Virus-III, a former name for HIV, now no longer in use.

immune system: A combination of cells and proteins that resist infection and other foreign substances in the body, including viruses and bacteria.

immunity: The condition of a living organism whereby it resists and overcomes infection and disease.

immunodeficiency: Any decrement in the ability of the immune system to respond appropriately to foreign substances or organisms.

immunoglobulin: Antibody-rich preparations administered to individuals after exposure to certain infectious agents to reduce the likelihood of developing infection.

immunocompetent: Having a normal functioning immune system.

immunosuppressed: See immunodeficiency.

incidence rate: The number of new cases of a disease that occurs per the population at risk, often reported per year and per 100,000 people.

incubation period: The period between infection and the onset of symptoms.

infection: The invasion of a host by organisms such as viruses, fungi, protozoa, or bacteria with consequent disease.

interferon: A protein formed by some cells after exposure to viruses that reduces viral replication; several types exist including alpha, beta, and gamma interferon.

interleukin-2: A protein derived from lymphocytes that promotes the growth of T lymphocytes and promotes the immune response of T cells.

intravenous (IV): Injected or delivered through a needle into a vein.

intravenous drug users: Individuals who inject substances into their bloodstream through a vein; also called injection drug users.

in vitro: A process occurring in the laboratory or other sites as opposed to occurring in the body.

isosporiasis: Infection by any member of the protozoan family of *Isospora*.

Isospora belli: A protozoan that occasionally causes disease of the small intestine and colon in humans, in AIDS patients infection leads to severe diarrhea.

Kaposi's sarcoma: A malignancy of the skin and lymph nodes that occurs frequently in AIDS patients; it usually appears as painless nodules and is an AIDS-defining illness.

Lymphadenopathy-associated virus (LAV): An early name for HIV and no longer in use.

lesbian: A female homosexual.

lymph: A clear fluid collected from tissues throughout the body and contained in lymph vessels.

lymphadenopathy: disease affecting a lymph node, often producing enlargement of the node.

lymph node: Tissues intercalated in lymph vessels; lymph nodes contain large numbers of various types of lymphocytes and are the site of a variety of immunological phenomena.

lymphocyte: A white blood cell found in blood and other body fluids and tissues; it participates in the immune response.

lymphoma: Any malignant tumor of the lymphatic tissues.

macrophage: A white blood cell that participates in the immune response and is infected by HIV.

meningitis: Any inflammation of the membranes lining the spinal cord and brain.

microbe: A microscopic organism.

microorganism: An organism of microscopic scale; synonymous with microbe.

molluscum contagiosum: A viral skin disease that affects the face and anogenital area; it is sexually transmissible and often asymptomatic although in individuals with immune compromise the disease may be extensive and symptomatic.

monocyte: A large white blood cell that is a precursor of macrophages and is infected by HIV.

monogamy: Having only one sexual partner.

mortality: Death rate.

mucous membranes: The surfaces lining cavities and canals of the body that communicate with air, such as the mouth and anus.

multiple sclerosis: A neurological disease of unknown cause characterized by episodes of neurological dysfunction involving the brain and spinal cord.

murine: Of or related to the mouse.

***Mycobacterium avium-intracellulare*:** A species of Mycobacteria, a type of bacteria, that can cause severe and usually systemic disease in immunocompromised patients.

***Mycobacterium avium* complex:** Organisms belonging to the genus *Mycobacteria* (consisting of *M. avium*, *M. intracellulare* and other species).

nanometer: One billionth of a meter.

National Institutes of Health: A division of the United States Department of Health and Human Services located in Bethesda, Maryland and devoted to clinical and basic science research in public health and the disease of humans.

neuropathy: Any disease or dysfunction of the peripheral nerves.

neutropenia: The presence of abnormally low numbers of neutrophils in the circulating blood. Neutrophils are white blood cells important in the host defense against specific microorganisms.

Non-Hodgkins lymphoma: A type of lymphoma that is prevalent in AIDS.

nucleic acid: A compound found in all viruses and living organisms that carries genetic information; DNA and RNA are the two principal forms.

opportunistic: The quality of a pathogen to produce disease only when infecting an immunologically compromised host.

pandemic: An epidemic over a wide geographic area, usually worldwide.

pathogen: A microorganism capable of causing disease.

PCR: Polymerase chain reaction assay; an assay used to measure the amount of HIV virus in the blood.

persistent generalized lymphadenopathy (PGL): A distinct syndrome in HIV infection in which lymph nodes in diverse parts of the body enlarge chronically.

Phase I study: The first step of drug testing in humans; its goal is to assess the side effects of drugs in small numbers of patients.

Phase II study: The second step of drug testing in humans; its purpose is to establish the activity and dosing of a drug while expanding its safety profile.

Phase III study: A late step in investigating new drugs; its goal is to prove the safety and efficacy of a new compound.

placebo: A pharmacologically inactive substance, often used in studies to compare against clinical responses to pharmacologically active substances.

placenta: The blood-filled organ that connects the fetus by the umbilical cord to the uterine wall; it is the source of blood exchange between the mother and the developing fetus during pregnancy.

Pneumocystis carinii: An organism found widely in nature that causes severe lung disease in those with AIDS or other profound immunodeficiency.

pneumonia: A type of inflammation of the lungs usually associated with infection with a microorganism.

prenatal: Existing or occurring before birth.

prevalence rate: Frequency of a disease in a population, usually expressed as the number of cases per 100,000 population.

protein: Molecules found in all forms of life that are the principal components of all tissues.

prospective: Looking and observing forward through time.

protozoan: A one-celled organism of the animal kingdom containing many different species; some cause disease in humans especially in the setting of altered immunity.

quarantine: Any limitation of movement or isolation imposed on an individual to prevent the spread of contagious disease.

retrospective: Looking back through time after an event has already occurred.

retrovirus: A class of viruses that contain RNA as their genetic material and require the enzyme reverse transcriptase to generate a DNA copy of the RNA.

reverse transcription: The process by which viral RNA is converted to DNA.

risk group: A group of individuals sharing a common behavior or characteristic placing them at a risk for HIV infection that is higher than the general population.

RNA: A nucleic acid related to DNA that carries genetic information in some viruses and virus-like agents, but in more complicated organisms is an intermediary between DNA and protein.

seroconversion: The time at which antibodies are produced against HIV in an infected individual.

seropositivity: Synonymous with antibody positivity.

seronegativity: The absence of antibodies directed against HIV and indicative of no infection; synonymous with antibody negativity.

serum: The cell-free fluid of the bloodstream, such as that appearing in a test tube after blood clots.

simian immunodeficiency syndrome (SAIDS): An immunodeficiency syndrome with similarities to AIDS found in some macaques infected with SIV, a retrovirus related to HIV.

syncytia: A clump of HIV-infected cells fused into a single, large dying cell.

syndrome: A group of symptoms and signs, which when considered together, constitute or characterize a disease.

systemic lupus erythematosus: A disease of unknown etiology characterized by fever, muscle pains, joint pains, skin rashes, anemia, and low white blood cell counts; it affects connective tissue, as well as the kidneys, spleen, skin, heart and the nervous system.

T cell: A type of lymphocyte crucial to immunity and an essential element in cellular immunity directed against viruses, parasites, fungi, and malignant cells.

thrush: A fungal infection due to *Candida albicans* found in the mouth; it is characterized by white spots on the tongue and inner surfaces of the cheeks.

***Toxoplasma gondii*:** A protozoan found throughout the world; the causative agent of toxoplasmosis, a devastating disease of the nervous system and eyes in immunocompromised hosts.

United States Public Health Service: The federal agency concerned with improving the health of the nation through basic and clinical research.

vaccine: A preparation administered to induce immunity against a particular pathogen without causing severe infection and disease; vaccines are intended to induce immunity by generating antibodies and cellular immune responses against the potential pathogen.

varicella-zoster virus: The virus that causes chicken pox and herpes zoster (shingles) infections.

venereal: Pertaining to sexual intercourse.

viral load: The quantity of HIV, measured as viral particles per mL of blood or any other tissue.

virions: An individual viral particle.

Western blot: A test to diagnose HIV infection through detection of antibodies against the virus.

zidovudine: See AZT.

—REFERENCES—

All references are keyed to question number. Journal abbreviations appear at end of section.

1. What is AIDS?
CDC. MMWR 31 (1982): 507-514.
CDC. MMWR 30 (1981): 250-252.
CDC. MMWR 25 (1981): 305-308.
Fauci A, et al. Ann Intern Med 100 (1984): 92-106.
Gottlieb M, et al. N Engl J Med 305 (1981): 1425-1431.
Jaffe H, et al. Ann Intern Med 99 (1983): 145-158.

2. Is AIDS a new illness?
Krause R. Science 257 (1992): 1073-1077.
Letvin N, et al. PNAS 80 (1983): 2118-2722.
Marx P, et al. Science (1984): 1083-1085.

3. What is the evidence that HIV causes AIDS?
Coombs R, et al. J Infect Dis 174 (1996): 704-712.
Kaminsky L, et al. PNAS 82 (1985): 5535-5539
Levy J, et al. Science 225 (1984): 840-842.
Schechter M, et al. Lancet 341 (1993): 658-659.
Weiss RA. Science 260 (1993): 1273-1279.

4. What is normal immunity?
Tonegawa S. Sci Amer 253 (1985): 122-131.

5. What is an opportunistic infection?
Broder S, Merigan T, Bolognesi D (eds). Textbook of AIDS Medicine (Baltimore: Williams & Wilkins, 1994).

6. How does HIV decrease immunity?
Levy J. Microbiol Rev. 57 (1993): 183-289.
McCune J. Cell 64 (1991): 351-363.
Tonegawa S. Sci Amer 253 (1985): 122-131.

7. What type of virus is HIV?
Wong-Staal F. In: B.N. Fields et al. (ed.) Fundamental Virology,
2nd ed, (New York: Raven Press, 1991), 709-723.

8. What are retroviruses?
Coffin J. In: B.N. Fields et al. (ed.) Fundamental Virology, 2nd
ed, (New York: Raven Press, 1991), 645-708.

9. How did HIV originate?
Gao F, et al. Nature 358 (1992): 495-499.
Koprowski H. Science 257 (1992): 1026-1027.
Kyle W. Lancet 339 (1992): 600-601.

10. Can monkey retroviruses infect humans?
CDC. MMWR 36 (1992): 678-681.
Gao F, et al. Nature 358 (1992): 495-499.
Khabbaz R, et al. Lancet 340 (1992): 271-273.

11. What is the definition of AIDS?
CDC. MMWR 41 (1992): 1-19.
CDC. MMWR 36 suppl 1 (1987): 1S-15S.
CDC. MMWR 31 (1982): 504-514.

12. What is the natural history of infection with HIV?
Saag M. In AIDS: Biology, Diagnosis, Treatment, and
Prevention (4th ed). Ed by Devita V, Hellman S, Rosenberg
S. (Philadelphia: Lippincott-Raven, 1997), 203-213.

13. What is the incubation period for AIDS?
Alcabes P, et al. Ann Epidemiology 4 (1994): 17-26.
Moss A, et al. BMJ 296 (1988): 745-750.
Phillips A, et al. Lancet 337 (1991): 389-392.
Phillips A, et al. J Acquir Immune Defic Syndr 4 (1991):
970-975.
Rosenberg P, et al. J Acquir Immune Defic Syndr 4 (1991):
392-401.
Taylor J, et al. J Acquir Immune Defic Syndr 4 (1991): 69-75.

14. How long will persons remain asymptomatic after infection?
CDC. MMWR 35 (1986): 448-451.
CDC. MMWR 34 (1985): 573-575.
Coombs R, et al. J Infect Dis 174 (1996): 704-12.
Daley C, et al. N Engl J Med 326 (1992): 231-235.
Hessol N, et al. Am J Epidemiol 30 (1989): 1167-1175.
Kaplan J, et al. J Acquir Immune Defic Syndr 5 (1992): 565-570.
Learmont J, et al. Lancet 340 (1992): 863-867.
Lemp G, et al. JAMA 263 (1990): 1497-1501.
Melbye M, et al. Ann Intern Med 104 (1986): 496-500.
Valle S, et al. Lancet 1 (1985): 301-304.

15. What are the different stages of HIV infection?
CDC. MMWR 41 (1992): 1-19.
CDC. MMWR 36 (1988): 821.
Redfield R, et al. N Engl J Med 314 (1986): 131-132.
Saag M. In: AIDS: Biology, Diagnosis, Treatment, and Prevention (4th ed). Ed by DeVita V, Hellman S, Rosenberg S. (Philadelphia: Lippincott-Raven, 1997), 203-213.

16. What is acute HIV infection?
Carne C, et al. Lancet 2 (1985): 1206-1208.
Cooper D, et al. Lancet 1 (1985): 537-540.
Tindall B, et al. Arch Intern Med 148 (1988): 945-949.

17. What are symptoms associated with acute HIV infection?
Kinloch De Loees S, et al. N Engl J Med 333 (1995): 408-413.
Schaker T, et al. Ann Intern Med 125 (1996): 257-264.
Tindall B, Cooper D. AIDS Pub Pol J 5 (1991): 1-14.

18. What are some of the early symptoms following acute infection?
Cooper G, Jeffers D. J Gen Intern Med 3 (1988): 525-532.
Fauci A, et al. Ann Intern Med 102 (1985): 800-813.
Gold J, et al. Medicine 64 (1985): 203-213.
Haverkos H. J Infect Dis 152 (1985): 1095.
Metroka C, et al. Ann Intern Med 99 (1983): 585-591.
Osmond D, et al. N Engl J Med 317 (1987): 246.
Volberding P. J Acquir Immune Defic Syndr 2 (1989): 421-425.

19. What are the symptoms of AIDS?
DeVita V, et al (eds). AIDS: Bilogy, Diagnosis, Treatment and
Prevention (4th ed). (Philadelphia: Lippincott-Raven, 1997),
203-443.

20. What role do opportunistic infections play in AIDS?
CDC. MMWR 41 (1992): 1-11.
Phair J, et al. N Engl J Med 322 (1990): 161-165.
Safrin S, Wofsy C, Sande M. The AIDS Knowledge Base.
Ed. by Cohen P, Sande M, Volberding P. (Waltham:
Medical Publishing, 1994).
Sattler F, et al. Ann Intern Med 109 (1988): 280-286.

21. What is oral hairy leukoplakia?
Maden C, et al. J Aquir Immune Def Syndr 7 (1994): 972-77.
Quinn T. "International AIDS." In Infectious Diseases. Ed. by
Gorbach S, et al. (Philadelphia: W.B.Saunders, 1992), 918-31.
Walling D, et al. J Virol 12 (1994): 7918-7926.

22. What is Pneumocystis carnii?
Kovacs J, Masur H. Infect Dis Clin North Am 14 (1992):
1003-1009.
Schwartlander B, et al. AIDS Pub Pol J 6 (1992): 413-420.
Simonds RJ, et al. Clin Infect Dis 24 supp 1 (1995): S44-S48

23. What is Kaposi's sarcoma?
Archibald C, et al. Epidemiology 3 (1992): 203-209.
Gao SJ, et al. N Engl J Med 335 (1996): 233-241.
Northfelt D, et al. Hematol Oncol Clin North Am 5 (1991):
297-310.

24. What is toxoplasmosis?
Barbaro G, et al. Scand J Infect Dis 27 (1995): 613-617.
Israelski DM, et al. J Acquir Immun Def Syndr 6 (1993):
414-418.
Luft B, et al. N Engl J Med 329 (1993): 995-1000.
Porter S, Sande M. N Engl J Med 327 (1992): 1643-1648.

25. What is Mycobacterium avium complex (MAC)?

Havlir DV, et al. N Engl J Med 335 (1996): 392-398.

Nightingale SD, et al. J Infect Dis 165 (1992): 1082-1085.

Shafran SD, et al. N Engl J Med 335 (1996): 377-383.

Pierce M, et al. N Engl J Med 335 (1996): 384-391.

26. What is candidiasis?

Crislip, et al. "Candida albicans and Related Species." In
Infectious Diseases. Ed. by Gorbach S, et al. (Philadelphia:
W.B.Saunders, 1992): 1887-1894.

Leport C, et al. J Infect Dis 173 (1996): 91-97.

Opravil M, et al. Clin Infect Dis 20 (1995): 531-541.

Oksenhendler E, et al. AIDS 8 (1994): 483-487.

27. What are the other fungal infections that affect AIDS patients?

Grayhill J. "Cryptococcus neoformans." Wheat L. "Histoplasma
capsulatum." In Infectious Diseases. Ed. by Gorbach S, et al.
(Philadelphia: W.B.Saunders, 1992), 1895-1898, 1905-1912.

Pinner RW, et al. Clin Infect Dis 21 (1995): S103-S107.

28 & 29. What is cryptosporidosis? What is isosporiasis?

Juranek DD. Clin Infect Dis 21 supp 1 (1995): S57-S61.

Mannheimer S, Soave R. Infect Dis Clin N Amer 8 (1994):
483-498.

Soave R, et al. "Crptosporidium, Isospora, Dientamoeba." In
Infectious Diseases. Ed. by Gorbach S, et al. (Philadelphia:
W.B.Saunders, 1992), 1328-1343.

30. What is zoster?

Glesby MJ, et al. Clin Infect Dis 21 (1995): 370-375.

Grose C, et al. "Varicella-Zoster Virus." In Infectious Diseases.
Ed. by Gorbach S, et al. (Philadelphia: W.B. Saunders, 1992),
1711-1714.

31. What is herpes simplex?

Oxman M. "Genital Herpes." In Infectious Diseases. Ed by
Gorbach S, et al. (Philadelphia: W.B.Saunders, 1992), 828-44.

Stewart JA, et al. Clin Infect Dis 21 supp 1 (1995): S114-S120.

32. What is cytomegalovirus?

Cheeseman S. "Cytomegalovirus." In Infectious Diseases. Ed. by Gorbach S, et al. (Philadelphia: W.B.Saunders, 1992), 1715-1720.

Spector S, et al. N Engl J Med 334 (1996): 1491-1497.

33. What is progressive multifocal leukoencephalopathy?

Holman, et al. Neurology 41 (1991): 1733-1736.

McArthur J. In: Infectious Diseases. Ed. by Gorbach S, et al. (Philadelphia: W.B.Saunders, 1992), 956-973.

34. What are non-Hodgkin's lymphomas?

Boyle M, et al. J Acquir Immune Defic Syndr 6 suppl 1 (1993): S5-S9.

35. What is cervical dysplasia?

Baker DA. AIDS Res Hum Retroviruses 10 (1994): 935-938.

Schafer A, et al. Am J Obstet Gynecol 164 (1991): 593-599.

Vernon SD, et al. Clin Infect Dis 21 supp 1 (1995): S121-S124.

36. What cases the wasting syndrome in patients with HIV infection?

Grunfeld C, Feingold K. N Engl J Med 327 (1992): 329-337.

Macallan DC, et al. N Engl J Med 333 (1995): 83-88.

Weinroth SE, et al. Infect Agents Dis 4 (1995): 76-94.

37. Can HIV-infected persons reduce the risk of acquiring opportunistic infections?

CDC. MMWR 44 (1995): 1-25.

Jewett J, Hecht F. JAMA 269 (1993): 1144-1153.

38. Can a person have an opportunistic infection and a low CD4 cell count without actually being HIV infected?

CDC. MMWR 41 (1992): 541-545.

CDC. MMWR 41 (1992): 578-579.

Fauci A, et al. N Engl J Med 328 (1993): 428-430.

Smith D. N Engl J Med 328 (1993): 373-379.

39. What symptoms of AIDS are not caused by opportunistic infections?
Bacellar H, et al. Neurology 44 (1994): 1892-1900.
Gendelman H, et al. AIDS 3 (1989): 475-495.
Gonda M, et al. Science 227 (1985): 173-177.
Ho D, et al. Ann Intern Med 111 (1989): 400-410.
Mintz M. Adv Neuroimmunol 4 (1994): 207-221.

40. Does HIV infection differ in women and men?
Brettle R, Leen C. AIDS Pub Pol J 5 (1991): 1283-1292.
CDC. MMWR 34 (1985): 721-726, 731-732.
Chaisson R, et al. N Engl J Med 333 (1995): 751-756.
Weinberg E. Rev Infect Dis 6 (1984): 814-831.

41. How does HIV affect children?
Burgard M, et al. N Engl J Med 327 (1992): 1192-1197.
Cassol S, et al. J Acquir Immune Defic Syndr 5 (1992): 13-119.
Landesman S, et al. JAMA 266 (1991): 3443-3446.
Marion R, et al. Am J Dis Child 140 (1986): 638-640.
Pizzo P. J Infect Dis 161 (1990) 316-325.
Pizzo P, Wilfert M. J Acquir Immune Defic Syndr Hum Retrovirol 8 (1995): 30-44.
Scott G. J Acquir Immune Defic Syndr 4 (1991): 109-115.

42. Who gets AIDS?
Centers for Disease Control and Prevention, Atlanta GA, 1996.
Holmberg S. Am J Public Health 86 (1996): 642-654.

43. What are principle routes of HIV transmission?
Chlebowski R. Nutr Cancer 7 (1985): 85-91.
Connor E, et al. N Engl J Med 331 (1994): 1173-1180.
Dean M, et al. Science 273 (1996): 1856-1862.
Lackritz E, et al. N Engl J Med 333 (1995): 1721-1725.
Liu R, et al. Cell 86 (1996): 367-377.
Real F, et al. Am J Med 80 (1986): 119-122.
Shafer R, et al. Lancet 1 (1985): 934-935.

44. Which body fluids contain HIV?

Fazakerly J, Webb H. Lancet 2 (1985): 891-892.

Groopman J, et al. Science 226 (1984): 447-449.

Krieger J, et al. J Infect Dis 163 (1991): 386-388.

Lifson A. JAMA 259 (1988): 1353-1356.

Rasheed S, et al. Am J Obstet Gynecol 175 (1996): 122-129.

Vogt M, et al. Lancet 1 (1986): 525-527.

Zagary D, et al. Science 226 (1984): 449-451.

45. How is HIV spread through sexual intercourse? Are women more susceptible to HIV infection from intercourse than men?

Calabrese L, Gopalakrishna L. N Engl J Med 314 (1986): 987.

CDC. MMWR 34 (1985) 561-563.

Hamed K, et al. J Infect Dis 167 (1993): 798.

Hayes R, et al. J Trop Med Hyg 98 (1995): 1-8.

Redfield A, et al. JAMA 254 (1985): 2094-2096.

Vogt M, et al. Lancet 1 (1986): 525-527.

Wofsy C, et al. Lancet 1 (1986): 527-529.

46. When does semen first contain HIV?

Archibald C, et al. Epidemiology 3 (1992): 203-209.

Krieger J, et al. J Infect Dis 163 (1991): 386-388.

Mascola L, Guinan M. N Engl J Med 314 (1986): 1354-1359.

Northfelt D, et al. Hematol Oncol Clin North Am 5 (1991): 297-310.

Stewart G, et al. Lancet 2 (1985): 581-584.

Tindall B, et al. AIDS Pub Pol J 6 (1992): 949-952.

47. What is the risk to heterosexuals of acquiring HIV infection?

Catania J, et al. Am J Public Health 85 (1995): 1492-1499.

Catania J, et al. Science 258 (1992): 1101-1106.

Centers for Disease Control and Prevention, Atlanta GA, 1996.

Lauver D, et al. J Obstet Gynecol Neonatal Nurs 24 (1995): 33-39.

48. What is the risk of HIV infection per episode of vaginal intercourse with an infected partner?

de Xincenzi I. N Engl J Med 331 (1994): 341-346.

Mastro T, et al. Lancet 343 (1994): 204-207.

Nicolosi A, et al. Epidemiology 5 (1994): 570-575.

49. What are the risks for wider spread of HIV in the heterosexual community?

Blower S. J Acquir Immune Defic Syndr 3 (1990): 763-772.

Mayer KH, Anderson DJ. Infect Agents Dis 4 (1995): 273-284.

Mhalu FS, Lyamuya E. East Afr Med J 73 (1996): 13-19.

50. How is HIV transmitted by homosexual intercourse?

Amerongen H, et al. J Acquir Immune Defic Syndr 4 (1991): 760-765.

Moss A, et al. Am J Epidemiol 125 (1987): 1035-1047.

Ostrow DG, et al. Am J Epidemiol 142 (1995): 875-883.

51. Are lesbians at risk for HIV infection?

Lemp G, et al. Am J Public Health 85 (1995): 1549-1552.

Petersen L, et al. J Acquir Immune Defic Syndr 5 (1992): 853-855.

52. Why do homosexual men form a large percentage of all AIDS cases?

Auerbach D, et al. Am J Med 78 (1984): 487-492.

Biggar R, et al. JAMA 231 (1984): 1441-1446.

CDC. MMWR 36 (1987): 137-140.

Glauser M, et al. Eur J Clin Microbiol 3 (1984): 55-58.

Goedert J, et al. Lancet 2 (1984): 711-716.

Kingsley L, et al. Lancet 1 (1987): 345-349.

Lifson A, et al. Am J Public Health 80 (1990): 1509-1511.

Mayer K, et al. Am J Med 80 (1986): 357-363.

Melbye M, et al. BMJ 289 (1984): 573-557.

Polk B, et al. N Engl J Med 316 (1987): 61-66.

Rozenbaum W, et al. Lancet 1 (1988): 1395.

Stewart G, et al. Lancet 2 (1985): 581-584.

Winkelstein W, et al. JAMA 257 (1987): 321-325.

53. Can HIV be transmitted via oral sex?

Baba T, et al. Science 272 (1996): 1486-1489.

Ho D, et al. Science 226 (1984): 451-453.

Lifson A, et al. Am J Public Health 80 (1990): 1509-1511.

Schacker T, et al. Ann Intern Med 125 (1996): 257-264.

Tindall B, et al. AIDS Pub Pol J 6 (1992): 949-952.

54. How is HIV transmitted via blood?

Blanche S, et al. N Engl J Med 320 (1989): 1643-1648.

Cowan M, et al. Pediatrics 73 (1984): 382-386.

Des Jarlais D, et al. Ann Intern Med 103 (1985): 755-759.

55. What is the risk of being infected with HIV via a blood transfusion?

CDC. MMWR 36 (1988): 833-845.

Cumming P, et al. N Engl J Med 321 (1989): 941-946.

Lackritz E, et al. N Engl J Med 333 (1995): 1721-1725.

The National Blood Resource Education Program Expert Panel.
    JAMA 263 (1990): 414-417.

Schreiber G, et al. N Engl J Med 334 (1996): 1685-1690.

Weiss S, et al. JAMA 254 (1985): 221-225.

56. Who should not donate blood?

Centers for Disease Control and Prevention, Atlanta GA.

57. Do other blood products transmit HIV?

CDC. MMWR 33 (1984): 685-687.

CDC. MMWR 35 (1986): 231-233.

CDC. MMWR 43 (1985): 489-491.

Cuthbertson B, et al. J Infect 15 (1987): 125-133.

Francis D, et al. JAMA 256 (1986): 869-872.

Sugg U, et al. Transfusion 27 (1987): 115.

58. How do IV drugs figure in the transmission of HIV?

Centers for Disease Control and Prevention, Atlanta, Georga.

Des Jarlais D, et al. AIDS Pub Pol J 6 (1992): 1053-1068.

Fordyce EJ, et al. AIDS 9 (1995): 605-610.

Friedland G, et al. Arch Intern Med 145 (1985): 1413-1417.

Hahn R, et al. JAMA 261 (1989): 2677-2684.

Schoenbaum E, et al. N Engl J Med 321 (1989): 874-879.

59. Can HIV transmission by intravenous drug users be reduced?
Cates W, Hinman A. N Engl J Med 327 (1992): 492-493.
CDC. MMWR 44 (1995): 684-685, 691.
Centers for Disease Control and Prevention, Atlanta, Georgia.
Des Jarlais D, et al. JAMA 274 (1995): 1226-1231.
Des Jarlais D, et al. AIDS Pub Pol J 6 (1992): 1053-1068.
Gostin L, et al. JAMA 277 (1997): 53-61.
Paone D, et al. Int J Addict 30 (1995): 1647-1683.
Watters J, et al. JAMA 271 (1994): 115-120.
Yancovitz S, et al. Am J Public Health 81 (1991): 1185-1191.

60. How is HIV passed to children and adolescents?
Blanche S, et al. N Engl J Med 330 (1994): 308-312.
Boyer PJ, et al. JAMA 271 (1994): 1925-1930.
CDC. MMWR 34 (1985): 721-726, 731-732.
Connor EM, et al. N Engl J Med 331 (1994): 1173-1180.
Dickover R, et al. JAMA 275 (1996): 599-605.
Gutman L, et al. Am J Dis Child 145 (1991): 137-141.
Landesman S, et al. N Engl J Med 334 (1996): 1617-1623.
Newell ML, Gibb DM. Drug Safety 12 (1995): 274-282.

61. Is HIV transmitted by breast feeding?
American Acadamey of Pediatrics Committee on Pediatric AIDS.
    Pediatrics 96 (1995): 977-979.
Black RF. J Am Diet Assoc 96 (1996): 267-274.
deMartino M, et al. AIDS Pub Pol J 6 (1992): 991-997.
Dunn D, et al. Lancet 340 (1992): 585-588.
Nicoll A, et al. AIDS Pub Pol J 4 (1990): 661-665.
Van de Perre P. Am J Obst Gyn 173 (1995): 483-487.
Van de Perre P, et al. N Engl J Med 325 (1991): 593-598.

62. Why are hemophiliacs at risk for HIV infection?
CDC. MMWR 37 (1988): 441-444, 449-450.
CDC. MMWR 34 (1985): 241-243.
CDC. MMWR 33 (1984): 589-591.
Evatt B, et al. Ann Intern Med 100 (1984): 499-504.
Koerper M, et al. Lancet 1 (1985): 275.
Kreiss J, et al. Am J Med 80 (1986): 345-350.
Levy J, et al. Lancet 1 (1985): 1456-1457.

Petricciani J, et al. Lancet 2 (1985): 890-891.
Ragni M, et al. Blood 70 (1987): 786-790.
Ragni M, et al. Am J Med 76 (1984): 206-210.

63. Do insects transmit HIV?

Castro K, et al. JAMA 259 (1988): 1338-1442.
CDC. MMWR 35 (1986): 609-612.
Chamberland M, et al. Ann Intern Med 101 (1985): 617-623.
Lifson A. JAMA 259 (1988): 1353-1356.
Mike L. Health Program, Office of Technology Assessment, U.S. Congress, Washington, D.C. (1987).

64. How can one reduce the sexual transmission of HIV?

CDC. MMWR 42 (1993): 589-591, 597.
CDC. MMWR 35 (1986): 152-155.
DeBuono B, et al. N Engl J Med 322 (1990): 821-825.
DiClemente RJ, Wingood GM. JAMA 274 (1995): 1271-1276.
Higgins D, et al. JAMA 266 (1991): 2419-2429.
Stryker J, et al. JAMA 273 (1995): 1143-1148.

65. What is safe sex?

Cohen PT, et al. In The AIDS Knowledge Base. Ed. by Cohen P, Sande M, Volberding P. (Waltham, MA: Medical Publishing, 1990).

66. What is the evidence that safe sex practices are effective?

CDC. MMWR 40 (1985): 613-615.
CDC. MMWR 3 (1984): 295-297.
DeBuono B, et al. N Engl J Med 322 (1990): 821-825.
Handsfield H. West J Med 143 (1985): 469-470.
Higgins D, et al. JAMA 266 (1991): 2419-2429.
Nelson K, et al. N Engl J Med 335 (1996): 297-303.
Winkelstein W, et al. Am J Public Health 77 (1987): 685-689.

67. Are condoms, diaphrams and spermicides effective in preventing HIV infection?

CDC. MMWR 37 (1988): 1925-1927.
de Vincenzi I. N Engl J Med 331 (1994): 341-346.
Guinan M. JAMA 268 (1992): 520-521.
Kreiss J, et al. JAMA 268 (1992): 477-482.

Perlman J, et al. J Acquir Immune Defic Syndr 3 (1990): 155
165.
Rietmeijer C, et al. JAMA 259 (1988): 1851-1853.

68. How can one minimize the risk of HIV transmission with condoms?
Faundes A, et al. Curr Opin Obstet Gynecol 6 (1994): 552-558.
University of California (Berkeley) Wellness Letter, December
1992.
Weir SS, et al. Genitourin Med 71 (1995): 78-81.

69. What is nonoxynol-9?
Bird K. AIDS Pub Pol J 5 (1991): 791-796.
Faundes A, et al. Curr Opin Obstet Gynecol 6 (1994): 552-558.
Kreiss J, et al. JAMA 268 (1992): 477-482.
Weir SS, et al. Genitourin Med 71 (1995): 78-81.

70. What other precautions reduce the risk of HIV infection?
CDC. MMWR 35 (1986): 152-155.
DeBuono B, et al. N Engl J Med 322 (1990): 821-825.
Higgins D, et al. JAMA 266 (1991): 2419-2429.
Hu D, et al. Bull World Health Organ 69 (1991): 623-630.
Wingood G, Di Clemente R. Am J Prev Med 12 (1996):
209-217.

71. Can HIV be transmitted through routes other than blood and sex?
CDC. MMWR 40 (1991): 21-21, 33.
CDC. MMWR 34 (1985): 533-534.
CDC. MMWR 34 (1985): 681-695.
CDC. MMWR 34 (1985): 681-695.
Fischl M, et al. JAMA 257 (1987): 640-644.
Friedland G, et al. AIDS Pub Pol J 4 (1990): 639-644.
Friedland G, et al. N Engl J Med 314 (1986): 344-349.
Gerberding J, et al. J Infect Dis 156 (1987): 1-8.
Yeung S, et al. J Infect Dis 167 (1993): 803-809.

72. What are the risks of HIV transmission in athletics?

Brown LS, et al. Ann Intern Med 122 (1995): 273-274.

Centers for Disease Control and Prevention, Atlanta, Georgia.

Mast EE, et al. Ann Intern Med 122 (1995): 283-285.

Goodman RA, et al. JAMA 271 (1994): 862-867.

Scott MJ, Scott MJ Jr. JAMA (letter) 262 (1989): 207-208.

The American Medical Society for Sports Medicine (AMSSM) and the Academy of Sports Medicine (AASM). Clin J Sport Med 5 (1995): 199-204.

World Health Organization, Geneva, Switzerland.

73. Are household members who care for AIDS patients at increased risk for HIV infection?

CDC. MMWR 36 suppl 2 (1987): 1S-18S.

CDC. MMWR 35 (1986): 76-79.

Kaplan J, et al. Pediatr Infect Dis 4 (1985): 468-471.

74. What are risks of transmitting HIV from a patient to a health care worker?

Centers for Disease Control and Prevention, Atlanta, Georgia.

Chamberland M, et al. Surg Clin North Am 75 (1995): 1057-1070.

CDC. MMWR 44 (1995): 929-933.

CDC. MMWR 36 (1987): 285-289.

Koenig S, et al. Am J Infect Control 23 (1995): 40-43.

O'Neill T, et al. Arch Intern Med 152 (1992): 1451-1456.

Shalom A, et al. J Occup Environ Med 37 (1995): 845-849.

75. What risks do patients have from HIV-infected physicians or other health care workers?

CDC. MMWR 42 (1993): 329.

CDC. MMWR 40 (1991): 1-9.

CDC. MMWR 40 (1991): 21-23.

Danila R, et al. N Engl J Med 325 (1991): 1406-1411.

Editorial. Lancet 340 (1992): 1259.

Lo B, et al. JAMA 267 (1992): 1100-1105.

76. What are appropriate precautions for health care workers to use with patients?

Barre-Sinoussi F, et al. Lancet 2 (1985): 721-722.

CDC. MMWR 37 (1988): 377-388.

CDC. MMWR 36 suppl 2 (1987): 1-18S.

Ho D, et al. N Engl J Med 313 (1985): 1606.

Hopkins C. Infect Dis Clin North Am 3 (1989): 747-761.

Jarvis R, et al. AIDS Law. (St. Paul: West Publishing, 1991).

Resnick L, et al. JAMA 255 (1986): 1887-1891.

77. What are adequate disinfection procedures for materials used by an HIV-positive patient?

FDA Medical Bulletin, March 3, 1993.

Sattar S, Springthorpe VS. Rev Infect Dis 13 (1991): 430-447.

78. Will mandatory testing of hospital patients protect hospital staff from infection with HIV?

Berglund C. Med Educ 29 (1995): 360-363.

Crosby C, Madden D. Internist 32 (1991): 18-19.

Wofsy C. Internist 32 (1991): 17-20.

79. How is HIV infection diagnosed?

Metcalf J, et al. In: DeVita V, et al (eds). AIDS: Biology, Diagnosis, Treatment and Prevention 4th ed. (Philadelphia: Lippincott-Raven, 1997), 177-196.

80. When is virus isolated from patients?

Coombs, et al. N Engl J Med 321 (1989): 1626-1631.

Dewar R, et al. J Infect Dis 170 (1994): 1172-1179.

Lafevillade A, et al. J Acquir Immune Defic Syndr 7 (1994): 1028-1033.

Perelson A, et al. Science 271 (1996): 1582-1586.

Saag M, et al. Nat Med 2 (1996): 625-629.

Stramer S, et al. JAMA 262 (1989): 64-69.

81. What is the antibody test used to diagnose HIV infection?

CDC. MMWR 36 (1988): 883.

CDC. MMWR 34 (1985): 477-478.

Sloand E, et al. JAMA 266 (1991): 2861-2866.

82. What is the role of the Western blot test?
Cooper D, et al. J Infect Dis 155 (1987): 1113-1118.
Davey R, et al. In AIDS: Etiology, Diagnosis, Treatment, and Prevention. Ed. by Devita V, Hellman S, Rosenberg S. (Philadelphia: J. Lippincott, 1992).
Imagawa D, et al. N Engl J Med 320 (1989): 1458-1462.
Sloand E, et al. JAMA 266 (1991): 2861-2866.

83 & 84. Indeterminate Western blot tests.
CDC. MMWR 41 (1992): 678-681.
CDC. MMWR 41 (1992): 814-815.
Celum C, et al. J Gen Intern Med 7 (1992): 640-645.
Courouce A. Lancet 2 (1989): 1330-1331.
Genesca J. Lancet 2 (1989): 1023-1025.

85. Are there any other kinds of HIV antibody tests available?
AIDS Alert 11 (1996): 94.
AIDS Policy Law 11 (1997): 9.
Emmons W, et al. J Infect Dis 171 (1995): 1406-1410.

86. What is the interval between infection and seroconversion?
Busch M, et al. Transfusion 35 (1995): 91-97.
CDC. MMWR 45 (1996): 181-184.
CDC. MMWR 39 (1990): 171-173.
Petersen L, et al. Transfusion 34 (1994): 283-289

87. Who should be tested for HIV antibody?
CDC. MMWR 44 (1995): 169-174.
Centers for Disease Control and Prevention, Atlanta GA.

89. What is the prevalence of the HIV antibody among various groups?
Centers for Disease Control and Prevention, Atlanta GA.

90. Are asymptomatic seropositive individuals infectious to other people?
Feorino P, et al. N Engl J Med 312 (1985): 1293-1296.
Krieger JN, et al. J Infect Dis 163 (1991): 386-388.

91. How can HIV infection be diagnosed in an infant?
Burgard M, et al. N Engl J Med 327 (1992): 1192-1197.
Lyamuya E, et al. J Acquir Immune Defic Syndr 12 (1996): 421-426.
Owens DK, et al. JAMA 275 (1996): 1342-1348.

92. Where can one receive HIV-antibody testing?
Centers for Disease Control and Prevention, Atlanta GA.
CDC. MMWR 41 (1992): 613-617.
CDC. MMWR 35 (1986): 284-287.
CDC. MMWR 34 (1985): 1-4.

93. Is there a role for a mass screening program?
CDC. MMWR 37 (1988): 461-463.
CDC. MMWR 35 (1986): 412-423.
Gostin L. JAMA 263 (1990): 2086-2093.
Janssen R, et al. N Engl J Med 327 (1992): 445-452.
Mauskopf J, et al. JAMA 276 (1996): 132-138.
Sperling R, et al. N Engl J Med 335 (1996): 1621-1629.

94. What issues may influence mandatory testing program?
Institute of Medicine. Confronting AIDS: Directions for Public Health, Health Care and Research. (Washington, DC: National Academy Press, 1986).
US Dept. of Health and Human Services, Public Health Service and CDC. "HIV counseling and testing in publicly funded sites: 1993-1994." Summary Report. June 12, 1996.
Wilfert C. N Engl J Med 335 (1996): 1678-1680.

95. Where does AIDS occur in the world?
Centers for Disease Control and Prevention, Atlanta, Georgia.
WHO. Weekly Epidemiological Report. 5 July 1996.
World Health Organization, Geneva, Switzerland.

96 - 99. International AIDS.
World Health Organization, Geneva, Switzerland.

100. What is the status of AIDS in Africa?

Biggar R. Lancet 1 (1986): 79-82.

Clumeck N, et al. JAMA 254 (1985): 2599-2608.

De Cock K, et al. Science 249 (1990): 793-796.

Mann J, et al. JAMA 255 (1986): 3255-3259.

Mertens TE, Low Beer D. Bull World Health Organ 74 (1996): 121-129.

Mhalu F, Lyamuya E. East Afr Med J 73 (1996): 13-19.

Nzilambi N, et al. N Engl J Med 318 (1988): 276-279.

Quinn T, et al. Science 234 (1986): 955-963.

Walraven G, et al. Trop Med Int Health 1 (1996): 3-14.

101. What is the Haitian link to AIDS?

Garris I, et al. J Acquir Immune Defic Syndr 4 (1991): 1173-1178.

Pape J, et al. N Engl J Med 309 (1983): 945-950.

Pitchenik A, et al. Ann Intern Med 98 (1983): 277-284.

102. Is HIV infection a major problem in prisons?

Brewer T, Derrickson J. AIDS Pub Pol J 6 (1992): 623-628.

CDC. MMWR 45 (1996): 268-271.

CDC. MMWR 411 (1992): 389-397.

103. What are the future prospects for HIV infection in the United States?

Brookmeyer R. Science 253 (1991): 37-42.

Centers for Disease Control and Prevention, Atlanta, Georgia.

CDC. MMWR 45 (1996): 121-124.

104. What are the projected costs of AIDS in the United States?

Centers for Disease Control and Prevention, Atlanta, Georgia.

Gable CR, et al. J Acquir Immune Defic Syndr Hum Retrovirol 12 (1996): 413-420.

Michaels D, Levine C. JAMA 268 (1992): 3456-3461.

Nicholas S, Abrams E. JAMA 268 (1992): 3478-3479.

105. What is the basis for developing drugs active against infection?

Corey L. In: G Mandell, et al. Principles and Practices of Infectious Diseases, 4th ed. (New York: Churchill Livingstone, 1995), 1267-1280.

106. What are the therapeutic approaches used to treat HIV infection?

De Clercq E. J Acquir Immune Defic Syndr 4 (1991): 207-218.

Schnittman S, Pettinelli C. In: DeVita V, et al (eds). AIDS: Biology, Diagnosis, Treatment and Prevention, 4th ed. (Philadelphia: Lippincott-Raven, 1997), 467-478.

107. What are therapeutic options for persons infected with HIV?

Collier A, et al. N Engl J Med 334 (1996): 1011-1017.

Deek SG, et al. JAMA 277 (1997): 145-153.

Graham N, et al. Lancet 1 (1991): 265-269.

Graham N, et al. N Engl J Med 326 (1992): 1037-1042.

Hamilton J, et al. N Engl J Med 326 (1992): 437-443.

Kahn J, et al. N Engl J Med 327 (1992): 581-587.

Katzenstein D, et al. N Engl J Med 335 (1996): 1091-1098.

Lagakos S, et al. JAMA 266 (1991): 2709-2712.

Schapiro J, et al. Ann Intern Med 124 (1996): 1039-1050.

Volberding P, et al. N Engl J Med 322 (1990): 941-949.

Yarchoan R, et al. In The Science of AIDS. (New York: W.H. Freeman and Co., 1989).

108. What is the most desirable treatment for HIV infection?

Collier A, et al. N Engl J Med 334 (1996): 1011-1017.

Ho D, et al. Nature 373 (1995): 123-126.

Markowitz M, et al. N Engl J Med 333 (1995): 1534-1539.

Perelson A, et al. Science 271 (1996): 1582-1586.

109. Is it possible to regenerate the immune system?

Giri N, et al. J Paediatr Child Health 28 (1992): 331-333.

Lane H, et al. Ann Intern Med 113 (1990): 512-519.

Lane H, et al. N Engl J Med 311 (1984): 1099-1103.

Lehman S. Nature 376 (1995): 204.

110. What is the evidence that antiretroviral therapy benefits patients?

O'Brien W, et al. N Engl J Med 334 (1996):425-431.

Saag M, et al. Nat Med 2 (1996): 625-629.

111. How do physicians decide to initiate antiretroviral therapy?

Broder S, et al. Ann Intern Med 113 (1990): 604-618.

Coombs R, er al. AIDS Clin Care 8 (1996): 1-8.

Katzenstein D, et al. N Engl J Med 335 (1996): 1091-1098.

Saag M, et al. Nat Med 2 (1996): 625-629.

Yarchoan R, et al. Ann Intern Med 115 (1991): 184-189.

112. What is the role of PCR and bDNA in the treatment of HIV infection?

Coombs R, et al. J Infect Dis 174 (1996): 704-712.

Ho D, et al. Nature 373 (1995): 123-126.

Japour A. J Int Assoc Physicians AIDS Care 2 (1996): 16-19.

Katzenstein D, et al. N Engl J Med 335 (1996): 1091-1098.

MacDougall D. J Int Assoc Physicians AIDS Care 2 (1996): 9-14.

Saag M, et al. Nat Med 2 (1996): 625-629.

113. What is the life expectancy for patients who receive zidovudine therapy?

Hammer S, et al. N Engl J Med 335 (1996): 1081-1090.

Lagakos S, et al. JAMA 66 (1991): 2709-2712.

114. Does HIV develop resistance to antiretroviral drugs?

Havlir D, Richman D. Ann Intern Med 124 (1996): 984-994.

Molla A, et al. Nat Med 2 (1996): 760-766.

Richman DD. Clin Infect Dis 21 Suppl 2 (1995): S166-S169.

Schapiro J, et al. Ann Intern Med 124 (1996): 1039-1050.

115. Does any therapy prevent infection in individuals recently exposed to HIV?

Callahan M, et al. Ann Emerg Med 20 (1991): 1351-1354.

CDC. MMWR 45 (1996): 468-480.

CDC. MMWR 44 (1995): 929-933.

Connor E, et al. N Engl J Med 331 (1994): 1173-1180.

Gerberding JL. Ann Intern Med 125 (1996): 497-501.
Sacks H, Rose D. J Gen Int Med 5 (1990): 132-137.

116. Is therapy beneficial in primary infection?
Kinloch-De Loes S, et al. N Engl J Med 333 (1995): 408-413.
Tindall B, et al. AIDS Pub Pol J 5 (1991): 477-484.

117. To what extent will antiretroviral therapy decrease transmission of HIV from a pregnant woman to her child?
CDC. MMWR 44 (1995): 1-15.
CDC. MMWR 43 (1994): 1-20.
Connor EM, et al. N Engl J Med 331 (1994): 1173-1180.
Dickover RE, et al. JAMA 275 (1996): 599-605.
Sperling R, et al. N Engl J Med 335 (1996): 1621-1629.
Wiznia AA, et al. JAMA 275 (1996): 1504-1506.

118. How can one estimate the prognosis of AIDS patients?
Moss A, et al. BMJ 296 (1988): 745-750.
Munoz A, et al. J Acquir Immune Defic Syndr Hum Retrovirol 8 (1995): 496-505.

119. Is the progression of HIV infection influenced by the strain of HIV that has infected the person?
Katzenstein D, et al. N Engl J Med 335 (1996): 1091-1098.
Learmont J, et al. Lancet 340 (1992): 863-867.
Verhofstede C, et al. AIDS 8 (1994): 1421-1427.

120. Who are "long-term non-progressors"?
Barker E, et al. PNAS USA 92 (1995): 11135-11139.
Cao Y, et al. N Engl J Med 332 (1995): 201-208.
Dean M, et al. Science 273 (1996): 1857-1862.
Levy J. AIDS 7 (1993): 1401-1410.
Levy J. Microbiol Rev 57 (1993): 183-289.

122. Do some adult groups differ significantly in their course of HIV infection from others?
Chaisson R, et al. 333 N Engl J Med (1995): 751-756.

123. How does the approach of AIDS patients to the terminal stages of their illness affect their treatment decisions?
Cote T, et al. JAMA 268 (1992): 2066-2068.
Steinbrook R, et al. N Engl J Med 314 (1986): 457-460.

124. Can children infected with HIV be vaccinated for other infectious diseases as is done with uninfected children?
CDC. MMWR 42 (1993): RR-4.
CDC. MMWR 38 (1989): 205-227.
Forrest J, Burgess M. Curr Opin Pediatr 8 (1996): 21-27.

125. Is it possible to develop a vaccine against HIV?
Bolognesi D, et al. AIDS Pub Pol J 4 suppl 1 (1990): s127-s128.
Graham B, Wright P. N Engl J Med 333 (1995): 1331-1339.
Hoth D, et al. Ann Intern Med 121 (1994): 603-611.
Letvin N. Curr Opin Immunol 4 (1992): 481-485.
Sabin A. PNAS 89 (1992): 8852-8855.
Schild G, Stott E. Vaccine 9 (1991): 779-781.

126. What is the process that leads to new drugs?
Food and Drug Administration, Rockville, Maryland.
Young F, et al. JAMA 259 (1989): 2267-2270.

129. How does the United States government fund HIV research?
Office of Budget, U.S. Public Health Service, Rockville, MD.

131. How can one evaluate alternative treatments for HIV infection?
McKean L. STEP Perspective, Feb 1993, 5-6.

132. How did HIV and AIDS initially impact public policy?
Senak M. HIV, AIDS and the Law (New York: Plenum, 1996).

133. Can results of an HIV-antibody test be given to public officials?
Senak M. HIV, AIDS and the Law (New York: Plenum, 1996).

134. Under what circumstances can sexual or other high-risk contacts of persons with HIV be notified by public officials?
CDC. MMWR 44 (1995): 202-204.
Gostin L. JAMA 261 (1989): 1621-1630.
Gostin L. JAMA 263 (1990): 1961-1970, 2086-2093.
Landis T. N Engl J Med 326 (1992): 101-106.
Wells K, Hoff G. Sex Trans Dis 22 (1995): 377-379.

135. Can life insurance companies require an individual to obtain HIV antibody testing as a condition for granting insurance?
Senak M. HIV, AIDS and the Law (New York: Plenum, 1996).

136. Can HIV antibody testing be used to deny employment?
Gostin L. JAMA 263 (1990): 1961-1970, 2086-2093.
Gostin L. JAMA 261 (1989): 1621-1630.
Landis T. N Engl J Med 326 (1992): 101-106.
Senak M. HIV, AIDS and the Law (New York: Plenum, 1996).

138. What role does quarantine play in reducing the spread of HIV?
Health and Public Policy Committee, American College of Physicians and the Infectious Diseases Society of America. Ann Intern Med 104 (1986): 575-581.

140. What are guidelines for HIV-infected children in school?
CDC. MMWR 41 (1992): 231-240.
CDC. MMWR 34 (1985): 517-521.
Gostin L. JAMA 263 (1990): 1961-1970.

141. What educational efforts are being made in public schools to decrease risk of HIV infection among adolescents?
CDC. MMWR 45 (1996): 760-765.
CDC. MMWR 44 (1996): 1-8.

143. What is the economic impact of AIDS in the United States?
Andrulis D, et al. JAMA 267 (1992): 2482-2486.
Green J, Arno P. JAMA 264 (1990): 1261-1266.
Hegarty J, et al. JAMA 260 (1988): 1901-1905.

Hurley S, et al. J Acquir Immune Defic Syndr Hum Retrovirol 12 (1996): 371-378.
Landesman S, et al. N Engl J Med 312 (1985): 521-524.
U.S. Department of Health and Human Services. Research Activities: Agency for Health Care Policy and Research. Washington, D.C., No. 155, 1992.

144. What are some of the ethical and social issues posed by the AIDS epidemic?

Berglund C. Med Educ 29 (1995): 360-363.
Brown J, Sprung C. Crit Care Clin 9 (1993): 115-123.
Connor S. Bull Pan Am Health Organ 23 (1989): 95-107.
Loue S, et al. J Law Med Ethics 23 (1995): 382-388.
Osborn J. AIDS Pub Pol J 3 suppl 1 (1989): s297-s300.
Razis D. Qual Assur Health Care 2 (1990): 353-357.
Rogers D, Osborn J. N Engl J Med 324 (1991): 1498-1500.

—JOURNAL TITLES—

AIDS Clin Care	AIDS Clinical Care
Adv Neuroimmunol	Advances in Neuroimmunology
AIDS Policy Law	AIDS Policy and Law
AIDS Pub Pol J	AIDS and Public Policy Journal
AIDS Res Hum Retroviruses	AIDS Research and Human Retroviruses
Am Fam Physician	American Family Physician
Am J Dis Child	American Journal of Diseases of Children
Am J Epidemiol	American Journal of Epidemiology
Am J Infect Control	American Journal of Infection Control
Am J Med	American Journal of Medicine
Am J Obstet Gynecol	American Journal of Obstetrics and Gynecology
Am J Pathol	American Journal of Pathology
Am J Public Health	American Journal of Public Health
Am J Prev Med	American Journal of Preventive Medicine
Ann Emerg Med	Annals of Emergency Medicine
Ann Intern Med	Annals of Internal Medicine
Arch Intern Med	Archives of Internal Medicine
BMJ	British Medical Journal
Bull Pan Am Health Organ	Bulletin of the Pan American Health Organization
Bull World Health Organ	Bulletin of the World Health Organization
Clin Infect Dis	Clinical Infectious Diseases
Crit Care Clin	Critical Care Clinics
Curr Opin Immunol	Current Opinion in Immunology
Curr Opin Obstet Gynecol	Current Opinion in Obstetrics and Gynecology

Curr Opin Pediatr	Current Opinion in Pediatrics
East Afr Med J	East African Medical Journal
Eur J Clin Microbiol	European Journal of Clinical Microbiology
Genitourin Med	Genitourinary Medicine
Hematol Onc Clinic North Am	Hematology and Oncology Clinics of North America
Infect Agent Dis	Infectious Agents and Disease
Infect Dis Clin North Am	Infectious Disease Clinics of North America
J Acquir Immune Defic Syndr	Journal of Acquired Immune Deficiency Syndrome
J Acquir Immune Defic Syndr Hum Retrovirol	Journal of Acquired Immune Deficiency Syndromes and Human Retrovirology
J Gen Intern Med	Journal of General Internal Medicine
J Infect	Journal of Infection
J Infect Dis	Journal of Infectious Diseases
J Int Assoc Physicians AIDS Care	Journal of the International Association of Physicians in AIDS Care
J Law Med Ethics	Journal of Law and Medical Ethics
J Obstet Gynecol Neonatal Nurs	Journal of Obstetric, Gynecologic and Neonatal Nursing
J Occup Environ Med	Journal of Occupational and Environmental Medicine
J Trop Med Hyg	Journal of Tropical Medicine and Hygiene
JAMA	Journal of the American Medical Association
Med Educ	Medical Education
Microbiol Rev	Microbiological Reviews

MMWR	Morbidity and Mortality Weekly Report
Nat Med	Nature Medicine
N Engl J Med	The New England Journal of Medicine
Nutr Cancer	Nutrition and Cancer
Pediat J Inf Dis	Pediatric Journal of Infectious Diseases
PNAS	Proceedings of the National Academy of Sciences USA
Rev Infect Dis	Reviews in Infectious Disease
Sci Amer	Scientific American
Sex Trans Dis	Sexually Transmitted Diseases
STEP Perspective	Seattle Treatment Education Project Perspective
Surg Clin North Am	Surgical Clinics of North America
Transfusion	Transfusion
West J Med	Western Journal of Medicine

Agencies and Organizations for HIV/AIDS Information

Several governmental agencies and private organizations supply information to individuals. Some of these groups are listed here.

Centers for Disease Control
CDC National AIDS Hotline
(800) 342-AIDS (2437 - English access)
(800) 344-SIDA (7432 - Spanish access)
(800) 243-7889 (Deaf access)

CDC National AIDS Information Clearinghouse
(Provides literature on HIV and AIDS.)
P.O. Box 6003
Rockville, MD 20849-6003
(800) 458-5231 (English & Spanish)
(800) 243-7012 (Deaf access)
(301) 217-0023 (international calls)
(301) 738-6616 Fax

Web site: http://cdcnac.aspensys.com
Email: aidsinfo@cdcnac.aspensys.com

The CDC is the most comprehensive service for HIV-related information in the United States. It provides a wide range of information to both individuals and to health professionals. Single copies of brochures, displays and reports are free. Multiple copies of certain documents can be obtained for a nominal fee.

AIDS Daily Summary; *Morbidity and Mortality Weekly Reports* (MMWR); and links to other AIDS-related Web and Gopher sites such as the National Library of Medicine, are available through the Web site (http://cdcnac.aspensys.com) or Email (aidsinfo@cdcnac.aspensys.com).

The Clearinghouse also operates several other HIV/AIDS information services:

AIDS Clinical Trials Information Service (ACTIS)
Provides information on experimental clinical trials that use drugs to treat HIV-related conditions.

(800) TRIALS-A, [or (800) 874-2572]
http://www.actis.org

AIDSNEWS Listserv
Provides automated mailing list sending Email to subscribers. This is a read-only mailing list and documents such as *AIDS Daily Summary*, selected *Morbidity and Mortality Weekly Report* articles, *CDC National Hotline Training Bulletins*, press releases from the FDA and National Institutes of Health as well HIV/AIDS fact sheets are available.

listserv@cdcnac.aspensys.com

CDC HIV/AIDS Prevention Newsletter
This newsletter is available from the CDC by written request.

1600 Clifton Road, MS/D-21,
Atlanta, GA 30333
or Email: lec4@oddhiv1.em.cdc.gov

CDC Division of HIV/AIDS Prevention

http://www.cdc.gov/nchstp/hiv_aids/dhap.htm

File Transfer Protocol (FTP)

Allows users to download files from host computer sites world wide, including current HIV/AIDS Surveillance Reports, AHCPR's clinical practice guidelines, and other documents.

Email: cdcnac.aspensys.com

Treatment Information

Provides current treatment information.

(800) HIV-0440 [or (800- 448-0440)]
http://www.hivatis.org
ftp://nlmpubs.nlm.nih.gov/aids/adatabases/drugs.txt

Business and Labor Resource Service

Provides educational materials.

(800) 458-5231.

OTHER SOURCES

AIDS Action Council

1875 Connecticut Ave. NW Suite 700
Washington, D.C. 20009
(202) 986-1300
(202) 986-1345 Fax
Email: HN3384@handsnet.org

AIDS Drug Information

http://www.pharminfo.com/

AIDS Treatment Data Network

611 Broadway, Suite 613
New York, NY 10012
(212) 260-8868
(800) 734-7104
http://www.aidsnyc.org/network
Email: AIDSTreatD@AOL.com

American Red Cross AIDS Education Office
8111 Gatehouse Road
Falls Church, VA 22042
(703) 206-7180
(703) 206-7673 Fax

Americans with Disabilities Act (ADA) Document Ctr.
(800) 514-0301
http://www.janweb.iedi.wvu.edu/kinder
(Information on the ADA, printed materials and access to other sites concerning disabilities, including HIV/AIDS.)

Department of Health and Human Services (DHHS)
http://www.os.dhhs.gov
(Central access point to DHHS data files, and government agencies such as Food and Drug Adminstration, Public Health Services, National Institutes of Health and Social Security Administration.)

Food and Drug Administration (FDA)
http://www.fda.gov
(Access to FDA activities, press releases, enforcement reports, drug approvals, Federal Register summaries, printed agency materials and *FDA Consumer* articles.)

Gay & Lesbian Medical Association
211 Church St., #C
San Francisco, CA 94114
(415) 255-4547
(415) 255-4784 Fax
Email: gaylesmed@AOL.com

Gay Men's Health Crisis
119 W. 24th St.
New York, NY   10011
(212) 807-6655
http://www.gmhc.org

ImmuNet Home Page
http://www.catalog.com/bwc/immunet/welcome.html
(Provides drug information.)

International Association of Physicians in AIDS Care
225 West Washington St., Suite 2200
Chicago, IL 60606-3418
http://www.iapac.org

Lambda Legal Defense and Education Fund
666 Broadway, Suite 1200
New York, NY 10012
(212) 995-8585
(212) 995-2306 Fax
Email: lldefny@AOL.com

Library of Congress
http://lcweb.loc.gov/homepage/lchp/html
(Access to catalogs and links to other government Internet sites
and resources.)

Names Project Foundation
310 Townsend St., Suite 310
San Francisco, CA 94107
(415) 882-5500
(415) 882-6200 Fax
http://www.aidsquilt.org
(Access to information regarding the AIDS Quilt, nationally,
regionally and local affiliates.)

National Association of People with AIDS (NAPWA)
1413 K Street, NW
Washington, DC 20005
(202) 898-0414
http://www.thecure.org

National Hemophilia Foundation
Soho Building
110 Greene St., Room 303
New York, NY   10012
(212) 219-8180
HANDI (Hemophilia and AIDS/HIV Network for the
Dissemination of Information: (800) 424-2634
(212) 966-9247 Fax)

National Institute of Allergy and Infectious Disease (NIAID)
http://www.niaid.nih.gov
(Access to AIDS related press releases, publications, grants and
contract information.)

National Institutes of Health (NIH)
http://www.nih.gov/
(Access to NIH health and clinical issues, NIH funded grants and
research activities.)

National Sexually Transmitted Diseases Hotline
American Social Health Association
P.O. Box 13827
Research Triangle Park, NC 27709
(800) 227-8922

National Women & HIV/AIDS Project
710 Eye St., SE
Washington, DC 20003
(202) 547-1155
womenaids@AOL.com

Project Inform's Treatment Information
1965 Market St., Suite 220
San Francisco, CA 94103
(415) 558- 8669
(800) 822-7422 (Hotline)
(415) 558- 0684 Fax
http://www.projinf.org
(Access to current treatment information for HIV disease.)

United States Public Health Service
Office of Communications
Hubert Humphrey BuildingRoom 721-H
200 Independence Ave., SW
Washington, D.C. 20201
(202) 690-6867

World Health Organization (WHO)
http://www.who.ch
(Access to WHO printed materials.)

Yahoo: AIDS/HIV
http://www.yahoo.com/Health/Diseases_and_Conditions/AIDS_
HIV/
(Access to 99 Web sites covering various HIV/AIDS categories.)

---

*Specialized scientific information is routinely reported in the
following journals which are often available in public and
medical libraries. These publications report both scientific and
therapeutic advances:*

*American Foundation for AIDS Research (AMFAR) AIDS/HIV
Treatment Directory*
Contains current HIV/AIDS treatment information, clinical drug
research protocols available nationwide, compassionate use and
expanded access programs, state drug assistance program
information, pharmaceutical drug assistance and other available
printed information.
Contact AMFAR at:
733 Third Ave., 12th Floor
New York, NY 10017-3204
(212) 682-7440
(800) 38-AMFAR subscription line
(212) 682-9812 Fax

Morbidity and Mortality Weekly Report (MMWR)
Contains information on the number of AIDS cases reported and
public health recommendations.
gopher://cwis.usc.edu/11/The_Health_Sciences_Campus/Periodi
cals/mmwr
http://www.cdc.gov/epo/mmwr/mmwr.html

Journal of the American Medical Association
http://www.ama-assn.org/journals/standing/jama/jamahome.htm
http://www.ama-assn.org/special/hiv//hivhome.

*Journal of the International Association of Physicians
in AIDS Care*

Lancet

Nature

The New England Journal of Medicine

Science

*Other general references found in specialized science libraries
that list journal articles for the biological and health sciences:*

Index Medicus

Current Topics

ASCATOPICS

The National Library of Medicine offers on-line computer
information on medical topics (MEDLINE) and AIDS-related
(AIDSLINE) topics. Information on access is available at:
(800) 638-8480
or http://www.nlm.nih.gov

Local information is generally available from the state public
health department serving a given municipality (see Appendix B).

HIV/AIDS Internet Resources

This list was compiled with the help of Pamela DeCarlo from the Center for AIDS Prevention Studies at the University of California in San Francisco. Sites are grouped into three categories: General, Medical and Reference.

GENERAL

AIDS Information for the Well-Informed
http://www.mediconsult.com/aids/
> *A site for health care professionals. Features journal club, support groups, drug and conference information.*

AIDS Research Information Center
http://www.critpath.org/aric/
> *A private, non-profit AIDS medical information service offering current, medically accurate information on AIDS treatment and research in plain English to anyone who requests it.*

AIDS Treatment Data Network (ATDN)
http://www.aidsync.org/network/index.html
> *A national clearinghouse for information about access to HIV treatments. Current information about how to gain access to drugs and treatments which are available through federal, state or pharmaceutical industry-sponsored programs plus New York-area HIV clinical trials.*

The Body
http://www.thebody.com/
> *A multimedia AIDS and HIV information resource featuring treatment, policy, prevention and community resources.*

CDC HIV/AIDS Treatment Information Site
http://www.hivatis.org/

CDC National AIDS Information Clearinghouse
http://cdcnac.aspensys.com

Center for AIDS Prevention Studies
http://www.epibiostat.ucsf.edu/capsweb
Focused on the prevention of HIV disease, contains fact sheets, information on its programs, and links to other sites.

Critical Path AIDS Project
http://www.critpath.org/
Extensive HIV/AIDS site. Includes full text copies of all ACTG AIDS clinical trial protocols.

European Information Center for HIV and AIDS
http://hiv.net
Information is available in either German, English, Italian, French or Spanish. Includes links to other international sites.

Family Health International
http://www.fhi.org

Immunet
http://www.immunet.org/

International Association of Physicians in AIDS Care (IAPAC)
http://www.iapac.org/index.html
Professional organization providing up-to-date drug and treatment information, CME courses, and clinician discussion groups.

JAMA HIV/AIDS Information Center
http://www.ama-assn.org/special/hiv/hivhome.htm
Site for the Journal of the American Medical Association includes journal club, expert advice, treatment information and searchable NLM database.

Medscape's AIDS Page
http://www5.medscape.com/Home/Topics/AIDS/AIDS.mhtml

National AIDS Treatment Advocacy Project
http://www.aidsync.org/natap/
Information on drug development, position papers, conference reports.

Project Inform
http://www.projinf.org/
An HIV information organization working on behalf of people living with HIV infection to keep them up-to-date on treatment, research and advocacy since 1985. Project Inform provides a free nationwide treatment hotline as well as Town Meetings presenting treatment information (monthly in San Francisco, and elsewhere by request). Information sheets and discussion papers are available by telephone and on the Net.

Advocacy and Policy

AIDS Action Council
http://www.thebody.com/aac/aacpage.html

AIDS Legal Referral Panel
http://www.lyb.com/high-brow/alrp-hp.html
Features information about life insurance and drug access.

Gay Men's Health Crisis
http://www.gmhc.org
Founded in 1981, this is the oldest and largest not-for-profit organization for AIDS/HIV in the United States.

National Association of People With AIDS Policy and Advocacy
http://www.thecure.org/napolicy.html

New York Academy of Medicine Action Alerts
http://www.aidsnyc.org/congress.html
Links to policy alerts, congressional e-mail addresses, and electronic activist sources.

Political Action Alerts from The Body
http://www.thebody.com/polact.html

Treatment Action Group
http://www.thebody.com/tag/tagpage.html

Caregiver Resources

CDC Guide to Caring for Someone with AIDS at home
http://www.hivatis.org/caring

Kairos Support for Caregivers
http://the-park.com/kairos/

Community Resources

AIDS Foundation Houston
http://www.powersource.com/afh/default.html

AIDS Prevention Project Seattle
http://www.metrokc.gov/health/apu/

Colordado AIDS Project
http://www.coloaids.org/

Nebraska AIDS Project
http://www.nap.org/

Project FIGHT
http://www.libertynet.org/~fight/
A community-based research initiative on AIDS in Philadelphia. This is a consortium of physicians and people living with HIV who have joined together to test potential treatments for HIV/AIDS and its complications.

Expert Advice

Dr. Joel Gallant from The Body
http://www.thebody.com/gallant/gallant.html

JAMA Expert Advice
http://www.ama-assn.org/special/hiv/advice/advihome.htm

Vanderbilt University HIV/AIDS Project
http://www.mc.vanderbilt.edu/adl/aids_project/help.html

Miscellaneous AIDS-Related Sites

ACT-UP New York
http://www.actupny.org
> *Home page for the HIV/AIDS activist group, AIDS Coalition To Unleash Power.*

AIDS Memorial Quilt
http://www.aidsquilt.org/

Artists With AIDS
http://www.artistswithaids.org

Mother's Voices
http://www.mvoices.org
> *Features information on how to talk to your children about AIDS.*

Safe Sex
http://weber.u.washington.edu/~sfpse/safesex.html
or
http://www.safersex.org

STOP AIDS
http://www.stopaids.org/

MEDICAL

Yahoo Medicine Listings
http://www.yahoo.com/Health/Medicine/

Alternative Medicine

ATDN's Alternative Treatments
http://www.aidsnyc.org/network/altx.html

Bastyr University AIDS Research Center
http://www.bastyr.edu/research/recruit.html

Clinical Trials

AIDS Clinical Trials Information from the CDC
http://www.actis.org/

AIDS Clinical Trials Unit at Washington University
http://www.id.wustl.edu/~actu/

CenterWatch Clinical Trials List
http://www.centerwatch.com/

Critical Path AIDS Project Trials List
http://www.critpath.org/trials.htm

The Network: Clinical Trials in New York Area
http://www.aidsync.org/network/trials.html

Trials Search: California HIV Clinical Trials
http://galen.library.ucsf.edu/aids/

Conferences

Conference Listings from IAPAC
http://www.iapac.org/conferences/conflist.html

Drugs

Antiviral info from The Body
http://www.thebody.com/treat/antivir.html

Antiviral Therapies from IAPAC
http://www.iapac.org/protidx.html

ATDN's Glossary of Drugs
http://www.aidsync.org/network/drugloss.html

Drug Database from PharmInfo Net
http://pharminfo.com/drugdb/db_mnu.html

FDA-Approved Drugs for HIV Infection and AIDS-Related Conditions
http://www.hivatis.org/fdachrt.html

FDA Center for Drug Evaluation and Research
http://ww.fda.gov/cder/drug.htm

Medical Sciences Bulletin
http://pharminfo.com/pubs/msb/msbmnu.html

Epidemilogy

CDC HIV/AIDS Surveillance Report
http://www.cdc.gov/nchstp/hiv_aids/statisti/hasrlink.htm
   AIDS and HIV cases in the United States by age, gender, race, risk factor and area.

Weekly Epidemiologic Review
http://www.who.ch/wer/issues.htm
   International AIDS cases.

Laboratories

HIV Sequence Database from the Los Alamos National Laboratory
http://hiv-web.lanl.gov/

WebPath
http://www-medlib.med.utah.edu/WebPath/webpath.html
The Internet Pathology Lab for Medical Education. Pictures of HIV, PCP, CMV and other infectious agents.

Treatment/Access to Treatment

AIDS Treatment Archive from The Body
http://www.thebody.com/atn/atnpage.html

AIDS Treatment Archive from Immunet
http://www.immunet.org/atn/

ATDN's Access Project
http://www.aidsnyc.org/network/access/index.html
State-by-state directory of medications available for HIV and AIDS through Medicaid, AIDS Drug Assistance Programs (ADAPs), and national pharmaceutical industry patient assistance/expanced access programs.

Infections and Complications from The Body
http://www.thebody.com/treat/oppinfs.html

Medscape's AIDS Page
http://www5.medscape.com/Home/Topics/AIDS/AIDS.mhtml

Opportunistic Diseases from IAPAC
http://www.iapac.org/diseases.html

Treatment Overview from The Body
http://www.thebody.com/treat/treatovr.html

REFERENCE

Fact Sheets

AIDS Treatment Data Network's Fact Sheets
http://www.aidsnyc.org/network/sf.html

National AIDS Treatment Information Project Fact Sheets
http://sfghaids.ucsf.edu/eduleve13factsheets.html

Government Resources

Centers for Disease Control and Prevention
http://www.cdc.gov/

CDC Division of HIV/AIDS Prevention
http://www.cdc.gov/nchstp/hiv_aids/dhap.htm

Department of Health and Human Services
http://www.os.dhhs.gov/

National Institutes of Health
http://www.nih.gov/

National Insitute of Allergy and Infectious Disease
http://www.niaid.nih.gov/

National Cancer Institute
http://www.nci.nih.gov/

National Institute on Drug Abuse
http://www.nida.nih.gov/

National Institute of Mental Health
http://www.nimh.nih.gov/

National Institute of General Medical Sciences
http://www.nih.gov/nigms/

National Library of Medicine
http://www.nlm.nih.gov/

NIH Division of Research Grants
http://www.drg.nih.gov/

United States Census Bureau
http://www.census.gov/

United States Public Health Service
http://www.os.dhhs.gov/phs/

Environmental Protection Agency
http://www.epa.gov/

National Academy of Sciences
http://www.nas.edu/

New York State Depratment of Health Home Page
http://www.health.state.ny.us/

Journals

British Medical Journal
http://www.tecc.co.uk/bmj/

Journal of the American Medical Association
http://www.ama-assn.org/special/hiv/library/libhome.htm

Morbidity and Mortality Weekly Report
http://www.cdc.gov/epo/mmwr/mmwr.html

Nature
http://www.nature.com

New England Journal of Medicine
http://www.nejm.org/

Science
http://science-mag.aaas.org/science/

Newsletters

AIDS Treatment News
http://www.thebody.com/atn/atnpage.html

HIV InfoWeb Database of Newsletters
http://www.jri.org/infoweb/treatment/library/readlist.htm

Positive Living from AIDS Project Los Angeles
http://www.apla.org/apla/positive-living.html

Research

National Library of Medicine AIDS Databases from JAMA
http://www.ama-assn.org/special/hiv/search/search.htm

—APPENDIX C—

State HIV/AIDS Programs

ALABAMA

AIDS Program Director
Alabama Department of Public Health
State Office Building, Room 662
434 Monroe Street
Montgomery, AL   36130
(334) 613-5366
(800) 228-0469

ALASKA

AIDS Public Health Representative
Department of Health and Social Services
3601 "C" Street, Suite 576
Anchorage, AK   99524-0249
(907) 269-8000
(800) 478-2437
(907) 562-7802 Fax

ARIZONA

Arizona Department of Health Services
431 North 24th Street
Phoenix, AZ   85008
(602) 230-5836
(800) 342-2437
(602) 230-5973 Fax

ARKANSAS

AIDS/STD Division
Arkansas Department of Health
4815 West Markham, Slot 33
Little Rock, AR   72205
(501) 661-2961

(800) 482-5400
(501) 661-2082 Fax

CALIFORNIA
Office of AIDS
California Department of Health Services
P.O. Box 942732
Sacramento, CA   94234-7320
(916) 323-7415
(800) 367-2437 (Northern California)
(800) 922-2437 (Southern California)
(916) 323-4642 Fax

COLORADO
Governor's AIDS Council
Colorado Department of Health
4300 Cherry Creek Drive S., DCEED-STD-A3
Denver, CO   80222-1530
(303) 692-2719
(800) 252-2437
(303) 782-5393 Fax

CONNECTICUT
Health Education and Intervention Division
Department of Public Health
Bureau of Community Health
410 Capitol Avenue, MS #11APV
Hartford, CT   06134-0308
(860) 509-7801
(800) 203-1234
(860) 509-7854 Fax

DELAWARE
State AIDS Activities, HIV/STD/AIDS Program
Delaware Health and Social Services, Division of Public Health
P.O. Box 637
Dover, DL   19903
(302) 739-3032
(800) 422-0429
(302) 739-6617 Fax

DISTRICT OF COLUMBIA
Agency for HIV/AIDS
Department of Human Services
717 14th Street, NW, Suite 600
Washington, D.C. 20005
(202) 727-2500
(202) 727-8471 Fax

FLORIDA
Office of Disease Intervention
Department of Health and Rehabilitative Services
1317 Winewood Boulevard
Building 2, Room 416
Tallahassee, FL 32399-0700
(904) 487-3684
(800) FLA-AIDS
(904) 487-1521 Fax

GEORGIA
STD/HIV Section
Epidemiology and Prevention Bureau
Department of Human Resources
Division of Public Health
2 Peachtree Street, N.W., 10th Fl., Rm. 400
Atlanta, GA 30303-3186
(404) 657-3100
(800) 551-2728
(404) 657-3133 Fax

HAWAII
STD/AIDS Program
Hawaii Department of Health
3627 Kilauea Avenue, Rm. 306
Honolulu, HI 96816-2399
(808) 733-9010
(808) 733-9015 Fax

IDAHO

STD/AIDS Program
Department of Health and Welfare
Bureau of Communicable Disease Prevention
450 West State Street, 4th Fl.
Boise, ID   83720-0036
(208) 334-6526
(208) 332-7346

ILLINOIS

AIDS Activity Section
Illinois Department of Public Health
160 N. LaSalle Street, 7th Fl. South
Chicago, IL   60601
(312) 814-4846
(800) 243-2438
(312) 814-4844 Fax

INDIANA

Indiana State Department of Health
Division of HIV/STD
2 N. Meridian St.
Indianapolis, IN   46204-3003
(317) 233-7851
(317) 233-7663 Fax

IOWA

STD/HIV Program
Iowa Department of Public Health
Lucas State Office Building, 4th Fl.
321 East 12th Street
Des Moines, IA   50319-0075
(515) 242-5838
(800) 455-2437
(515) 281-4529 Fax

KANSAS

Kansas Department of Health and Environment
Bureau of Disease Control
109 SW 9th Street, Suite 605

Topeka, KS   66612-1271
(913) 296-6173
(800) 232-0040
(913) 296-4197 Fax

KENTUCKY

HIV/AIDS Program
Department for Health Services
275 East Main Street
Frankfort, KY   40621
(502) 564-6539
(800) 654-AIDS
(502) 564-9865 Fax

LOUISIANA

HIV Program Office
Louisiana Department of Health and Hospitals
1600 Canal Street, Suite 900
New Orleans, LA   70112
(504) 568-7474
(800) 992-4379
(504) 568-7044 Fax

MAINE

HIV/STD Programs
Maine Bureau of Health
State House Station #11
Augusta, ME   04333-0011
(207) 287-5551
(800) 851-AIDS
(207) 287-6865 Fax

MARYLAND

AIDS Administration
Maryland Department of Health and Mental Hygiene
500 N. Calvert Street
Baltimore, MD   21202
(410) 767-5013
(800) 638-6252
(410) 333-6333 Fax

MASSACHUSETTS
Department of Public Health
AIDS Bureau
250 Washington Street, 3rd Fl.
Boston, MA   02108-4619
(617) 624-5300
(800) 750-2061
(617) 624-5399 Fax

MICHIGAN
HIV/AIDS Prevention and Intervention
Department or Health
3500 Martin Luther King Boulevard
P.O. Box   30035
Lansing, MI   48909
(517) 335-8468
(800) 872-AIDS
(517) 335-9611 Fax

MINNESOTA
AIDS/STD Prevention Services,
Disease Prevention and Control
Minnesota Department of Health
717 Delaware Street S.E., Box 9441
Minneapolis, MN   55440-9441
(612) 623-5143
(800) 248-AIDS
(612) 623-5743 Fax

MISSISSIPPI
Division of STD/HIV
Mississippi State Department of Health
P.O. Box 1700
Jackson, MS   39215-1700
(601) 960-7711
(800) 826-2961
(601) 960-7909 Fax

MISSOURI
Bureau of STD/HIV Prevention
Missouri Department of Health
1730 East Elm Street
P.O. Box 570
Jefferson City, MO   65102-0570
(573) 751-6141
(800) 359-6259
(573) 751-6417 Fax

MONTANA
Montana HIV/STD Project
Department of Public Health and Human Services
P.O. Box 202951
Helena, MT 59620-2951
(406) 444-3565
(800) 233-6668
(406) 444-2920 Fax

NEBRASKA
Communicable Disease Section
Nebraska Department of Health
301 Centennial Mall, South
P.O. Box 95007
Lincoln, NE   68509
(402) 471-2937
(800) 782-2437
(402) 471-6426 Fax

NEVADA
HIV/AIDS Program Office
Bureau of Disease Control and Intervention
Nevada State Health Division
505 E. King Street, Rm. 304
Carson City, NV   89710
(702) 687-4800
(702) 687-4988 Fax

NEW HAMPSHIRE
STD/HIV Program
New Hampshire Division of Public Health Services
Health and Welfare Building
6 Hazen Drive
Concord, NH   03301
(603) 271-4576
(800) 852-3345 x 4576
(603) 271-4934 Fax

NEW JERSEY
Division of AIDS Prevention and Control
50 East State Street, CN-363
Trenton, NJ   08625
(609) 984-5874
(800) 624-2377
(609) 633-2494 Fax

NEW MEXICO
HIV/AIDS/STD Bureau
New Mexico Department of Health
525 Camino de los Marquez, Suite 1 (Marquez Place)
Santa Fe, NM   87501
(505) 476-8451
(800) 545-2437
(505) 476-8527 Fax

NEW YORK
AIDS Institute
New York State Department of Health
Corning Tower, Rm. 342
Albany, NY   12237-0658
(518) 473-7542
(800) 541-2437
(518) 486-1315 Fax

NORTH CAROLINA
AIDS Care Branch
NC Department of Environment,
    Health and Natural Resources
P.O. Box 27687
Raleigh, NC   27611-7687
(919) 733-7301
(800) 342-2437
(919) 733-1020 Fax

NORTH DAKOTA
HIV/AIDS Program
North Dakota Department of Health
Division of Disease Control
600 East Boulevard
Bismarck, ND   58505-0200
(701) 328-2378
(800) 472-2180
(701) 328-1412 Fax

OHIO
HIV/STD Prevention Programs
Ohio Department of Health
Division of Prevention
Bureau of Infectious Disease Control
P.O. Box 118
Columbus, OH   43266-0118
(614) 728-9256
(800) 332-AIDS
(614) 644-1909 Fax

OKLAHOMA
HIV/STD Service
Oklahoma State Department of Health
1000 N.E. 10th Street and Stonewall
Oklahoma City, OK   73117-1299
(405) 271-4636
(405) 271-5149 Fax

OREGON
HIV Program
Oregon Health Division
800 NE Oregon Street, Suite 730
Portland, OR   97232
(503) 731-4029
(800) 777-2437
(503) 731-4082 Fax

PENNSYLVANIA
Pennsylvania Department of Health
Bureau of HIV/AIDS
Health and Welfare Building, Rm. 912
P.O. Box 90
Harrisburg, PA   17108
(717)-783-0479
(800) 662-6080
(717) 772-4309 Fax

RHODE ISLAND
Office of AIDS/STD
Rhode Island Department of Health
3 Capitol Hill, Rm. 105
Providence, RI   02908
(401) 277-2320
(401) 272-3771 Fax

SOUTH CAROLINA
STD/HIV Division
Health and Environmental Control
Box 101106
Columbia, SC   29211
(803) 737-4110
(800) 322-AIDS
(803) 737-3979 Fax

SOUTH DAKOTA
STD/HIV/AIDS Program
Communicable Disease Prevention and Control
South Dakota Department of Health

445 East Capitol
Pierre, SD   57501-3185
(605) 773-3737
(800) 592-1861
(605) 773-5509 Fax

TENNESSEE
STD/HIV Program - C.E.D.S.S.
Tennessee Department of Health
426 5th Avenue, North
Cordell Hull Building, 4th Fl.
Nashville, TN   37247-4911
(615) 741-7510
(800) 525-2437
(615) 741-3857 Fax

TEXAS
HIV/AIDS Health Resources Division
Texas Department of Health
1100 West 49th Street
Austin, TX   78756-9987
(512) 490-2515
(512) 490-2544 Fax

UTAH
Bureau of HIV/AIDS/TB and Refugee Health Prevention
Utah Department of Health
P.O. Box 142867
Salt Lake City, UT   84114-2867
(801) 538-6096
(800) 843-9388
(801) 538-6036 Fax

VERMONT
AIDS Program
Vermont Department of Health
P.O. Box 70
Burlington, VT   05402
(802) 863-7245

(800) 882-AIDS
(802) 863-7314 Fax

VIRGINIA
Bureau of STD/AIDS
Virginia Department of Health
P.O. Box 2448, Rm. 112
Richmond, VA   23218
(804) 786-6267/ (804) 371-7455
(800) 533-4148
(804) 225-3517 Fax

WASHINGTON
Infectious Disease & Reproductive Health
Washington State Department of Health
P.O. Box 47844
Olympia, WA   98504-7844
(360) 586-8344
(800) 272-AIDS
(360) 644-4239 Fax

WEST VIRGINIA
Division of Surveillance and Disease Control
1422 Washington Street, East
Charleston, WV   25301
(304) 558-5358
(800) 642-8244
(304) 558-6335 Fax

WISCONSIN
AIDS/HIV Program
Wisconsin Division of Health
1414 East Washington Avenue, Rm. 241
Madison, WI   53703
(608) 267-5287
(800) 334-2437
(608) 266-2906 Fax

WYOMING
Wyoming Department of Health
HIV/AIDS Prevention Program
Hathaway Building, 4th Fl.
Cheyenne, WY   82002
(307) 777-7703
(800) 364- 3104
(307) 777-5402 Fax

US TERRITORIES

GUAM
Department of Public Health and Social Services
Government of Guam
P.O. Box 2816
Agana, Guam   96910
(011) 671-735-7142
(011) 671-734-5910 Fax

MARSHALL ISLANDS
Ministry of Health Services
Republic of the Marshall Islands
P.O. Box 16
Majuro, Marshall Islands   96960
(011) 692-625-3355
(011) 692-625-3432 Fax

PALAU
Bureau of Health Services
P.O. Box 100
Koror, Palau PW 96940
(011) 680-488-1757
(011) 680 488-1725 Fax

PUERTO RICO
Program of AIDS Affairs and STDs
P.O. Box 71423
San Juan, PR   00936
(809) 274-5534/5532
(809) 274-5503 Fax

SAMOA
AIDS Program
Public Health Division
Department of Health
LBJ Tropical Medical Center
P.O. Box F
Pago Pago, AS   96799
(011) 684-633-4071
(011) 684-633-5379

VIRGIN ISLANDS
STD/HIV/TB Program
Virgin Islands Department of Health
48 Sugar Estate
St. Thomas, U.S.V.I.   00802
(809) 774-3168
(809) 777-4001 Fax

INDEX

—K—

—L—

ABOUT THE AUTHORS

Lyn Robert Frumkin is a graduate of the University of Washington where he obtained a combined M.D./Ph.D. degree. His postgraduate medical and research training has been at Stanford University, the University of California at Los Angeles, and the University of Washington. Dr. Frumkin is currently involved in research on AIDS and infectious diseases at Amgen, a biotechnology company in the Los Angeles area, and is on the faculty of the University of California at Los Angeles School of Medicine.

John Martin Leonard received his M.D. from The Johns Hopkins University. Dr. Leonard did postgraduate medical training at Stanford University and the National Institute of Allergy and Infectious Diseases, National Institutes of Health, where he conducted research on the molecular biology of HIV. He now directs the antiviral drug development section at Abbott Laboratories where he was instrumental in the development of HIV protease inhibitors.